C6/19

Ultrasonics in
Clinical Diagnosis

Ultrasonics in Clinical Diagnosis

Edited by

P.N.T. Wells, **D.Sc.,F.Inst.P.,F.I.E.E.**
Chief Physicist, Avon Area Health Authority (Teaching)

SECOND EDITION

CHURCHILL LIVINGSTONE
Edinburgh London and New York 1977

CHURCHILL LIVINGSTONE
Medical Division of Longman Group Limited

Distributed in the United States of America by
Longman Inc., 19 West 44th Street, New York,
N.Y. 10036 and by associated companies,
branches and representatives throughout
the world.

First Edition 1972
Second Edition 1977
    Reprinted 1979

ISBN 0 443 01644 5 (cased)
ISBN 0 443 01369 1 (limp)

Library of Congress Cataloging in Publication Data

Wells, Peter Neil Temple.
    Ultrasonics in clinical diagnosis.

    Includes bibliographies and index.
    1. Diagnosis, Ultrasonic. I. Title.
RC78.7.U4W46   1977   616.07'54   77- 1479

Printed in Great Britain by
T. & A. Constable Ltd., Edinburgh

Preface to the Second Edition

Ultrasonic diagnosis is used routinely in the investigation of many patients. During the five years since the publication of the first edition of this book, there has been an enormous increase in the number of ultrasonic instruments in use throughout the world. This growth is continuing. More and more doctors are coming to depend on ultrasonic diagnostic information, and patients are beginning to demand this method of examination.

This new edition aims to help in the training of the medical and paramedical staff who, in increasing numbers, are involved in ultrasonic diagnosis. It satisfies the needs of candidates for the Fellowship of the Royal College of Radiologists, and the examinations of the Society of Radiographers and the American Society of Ultrasound Technical Specialists. It should also be useful to medical specialists in other fields, hospital physicists and engineers in industry.

It has been an agreeable task for me to prepare for publication the contributions of my friends and colleagues. We have tried to incorporate suggestions made by reviewers of the first edition. I am grateful to my friends for having allowed me sometimes drastically to edit their manuscripts, so that their separate chapters, each a distinguished and definitive review, blend uniformly together.

My debt to the contributors is very great. But the publication of this book is also due to the help of many others. I cannot overemphasize the value of discussions which I have had with my colleagues, particularly Dr Peter Atkinson, Mr D.H. Follett, Dr Michael Halliwell, Dr R.A. Mountford, Professor A.E. Read and Dr J.P. Woodcock. Mrs Rosemary Cardwell and Miss Josephine Reynolds cheerfully deciphered the manuscript and did the typing. The staff of Churchill Livingstone have been both courteous and helpful. Last but not least, I am grateful for the encouragement of my wife and family.

1977   P.N.T. Wells

Contributors

Ian Donald, *M.B.E.,* M.D., B.A., F.R.C.S. (Glasgow), F.R.C.O.G.,
Department of Midwifery,
Queen Mother's Hospital,
Glasgow G3 8SH, U.K.

E.J. Giglio, O.D.,
Research Laboratories,
State College of Optometry,
122 East 25th Street,
New York,
NY 10010, U.S.A.

C.R. Hill, B.A., Ph.D., D.Sc., F. Inst. P., M.I.E.E.,
Department of Physics,
Institute of Cancer Research,
Sutton SM2 5PX, U.K.

F.G.M. Ross, B.A., M.B., B.Ch., B.A.O., D.M.R.D., F.R.C.R.,
Department of Radiodiagnosis,
Bristol Royal Infirmary,
Bristol BS2 8HW, U.K.

K.J.W. Taylor, B.Sc., M.D., Ph.D.,
Department of Radiology,
Yale University School of Medicine,
333 Cedar Street,
Newhaven,
CT 06510, U.S.A.

P.N.T. Wells, D.Sc., F. Inst. P., F.I.E.E.
Department of Medical Physics,
Bristol General Hospital,
Bristol BS1 6SY, U.K.

D.N. White, M.A., M.D., F.R.C.P.(C), F.A.C.P.,
Department of Medicine (Neurology),
Queens University at Kingston,
Ontario,
Canada K7L 3N6

Contents

9. Other ultrasonic investigations
F.G.M. Ross and P.N.T. Wells

PART III: BIOLOGICAL EFFECTS, INCLUDING THE POSSIBILITY OF HAZARD IN DIAGNOSTIC TECHNIQUES

10. Biological effects of ultrasound
C.R. Hill

PART I BASIC PRINCIPLES AND DIAGNOSTIC METHODS

1. Basic principles

P.N.T. WELLS

Ultrasonic diagnosis depends upon physical measurements of the interactions between ultrasonic waves and biological materials. An adequate knowledge of the basic physical processes involved in the generation, propagation and detection of ultrasonic waves is necessary for a proper understanding of ultrasonic diagnostic techniques. The contents of this chapter are intended to provide this background, in the simplest way.

1.1 FUNDAMENTAL PHYSICS

1.1.a. Wave motion

Ultrasound is a form of energy which consists of mechanical vibrations the frequencies of which are so high that they are above the range of human hearing. The lower frequency limit of the ultrasonic spectrum may generally be taken to be about 20 kHz*. Most diagnostic applications of ultrasound employ frequencies in the range 1–15 MHz.

Ultrasonic energy travels through a medium in the form of a *wave*. Although a number of different wave *modes* are possible, almost all diagnostic applications involve the use of *longitudinal* waves. The particles[†] of which the medium is composed vibrate backwards and forwards about their mean positions, so that energy is transferred through the medium in a direction parallel to that of the oscillations of the particles. The particles themselves do not move through the medium, but simply vibrate to and fro. Thus, the energy is transferred in the form of a disturbance in the equilibrium arrangement of the medium, without any bodily transfer of matter.

Ultrasound and other mechanical waves are quite distinct from electromagnetic waves. Electromagnetic waves consist of electric and magnetic fields, one field supporting and generating the other.

In an ultrasonic field, cyclical oscillations occur both in space and in time:-the simplest type is illustrated in Fig. 1.1. The oscillations here are continuous at constant amplitude, and the particles move with *simple harmonic motion*: when a particle is displaced from its equilibrium position it experiences a restoring force which is proportional to its displacement. This *direct proportionality* is the characteristic which distinguishes simple harmonic motion from other, more

---

*1 Hz (hertz) = 1 cycle per second. Thus, 1 kHz = 1000 cycles per second; 1 MHz = 1 000 000 cycles per second.

†A *particle* is a volume element which is large enough to contain many millions of molecules, so that it is continuous with its surroundings; but it is so small that quantities variable within the medium (such as pressure) are constant within the particle.

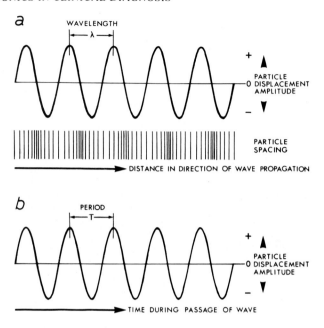

Fig. 1.1 Diagrams illustrating longitudinal wave motion. (*a*) Particle displacement amplitude and particle spacing at a particular instant in time in the ultrasonic field: these diagrams represent the distribution of the wave in *space*. (*b*) Particle displacement amplitude at a particular point in space in the ultrasonic field: this diagram represents the distribution of the wave in *time*.

complicated, disturbances. The *wavelength,* λ, is the distance in the medium between consecutive particles where the displacement amplitudes are identical; similarly, the wave *period, T,* is the time which is required for the wave to move forward through a distance λ in the medium. The *frequency, f,* of the wave is equal to the number of cycles which pass a given point in the medium in unit time (usually one second); thus,

$$f = 1/T \tag{1.1}$$

The wavelength and the frequency are related to the propagation velocity, c, by the equation

$$c = f\lambda \tag{1.2}$$

For example at a frequency of 1 MHz, the wavelength in water ($c = 1500$ m s^{-1}) is 1·5 mm.

These relationships apply strictly only to continuous waves of constant amplitude. Other types of disturbance (for example, pulsed waves) are not associated with a single frequency, and so λ and T are not constants (c is largely independent of frequency).

The velocity at which the energy is transferred through the medium is determined by the delay which occurs between the movements of neighbouring particles. This depends upon the *elasticity, K* (because this controls the force for a given displacement in the medium) and the *density,* ρ (which controls the acceleration for a given force within the medium) according to the equation

$$c = \sqrt{(K/\rho)} \qquad (1.3)$$

The velocities in soft tissues are closely similar. The velocity in bone is higher, whilst that in lung is lower. Velocities in various materials are given in Table 1.1.

Table 1.1.   Ultrasonic properties of some common materials, including biological tissues.

	Propagation velocity $(m\,s^{-1})$	Characteristic impedance $(10^6\,kg\,m^{-2}\,s^{-1})$	Attenuation coefficient at 1 MHz $(dB\,cm^{-1})$	Frequency dependence of attenuation coefficient
Air	330	0·0004	10	f^2
Aluminium	6400	17	0·02	f
Bone	2700–4100	3·75–7·38	3–10	f–$f^{1.5}$
Castor oil	1500	1·4	1	f^2
Lung	650–1160	0·26–0·46	40	$f^{0.6}$
Muscle	1545–1630	1·65–1·74	1·5–2·5	f
Perspex	2680	3·2	2	f
Soft tissues (except muscle)	1460–1615	1·35–1·68	0·3–1·5	f
Water	1480	1·52	0·002	f^2

1.1.b.   Behaviour at boundaries

When a wave meets the boundary between two media at normal incidence, it is propagated without deviation into the second medium. At oblique incidence (Fig. 1.2), the wave is deviated by *refraction* unless the velocities in the two media are equal. The relationship is

$$(\sin\theta_i)/(\sin\theta_t) = c_1/c_2 \qquad (1.4)$$

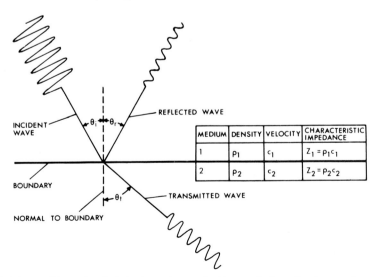

Fig. 1.2 Diagram illustrating the behaviour of a wave incident on the boundary between two media.

Sometimes a fraction of the incident wave is reflected at the boundary. In such cases, $\theta_i = \theta_r$, and the reflexion is said to be *'specular'*.

In any given medium, the ratio of the instantaneous values of particle pressure and velocity is a constant. This constant is called the *'characteristic impedance'*, Z, of the medium, and it is related to the density and velocity by the equation

$$Z = \rho c \tag{1.5}$$

Typical values of characteristic impedance are given in Table 1.1.

In a propagating wave, there are no sudden discontinuities in either particle velocity or particle pressure. Consequently, when a wave meets the boundary between two media, both the particle velocity and the pressure are continuous across the boundary. Physically, this ensures that the two media remain in contact. In each medium, however, the ratio of the particle pressure and velocity is fixed and equal to the corresponding characteristic impedance. If the characteristic impedances are equal, the wave travels across the boundary unaffected by the change in the supporting medium (apart from deviation by refraction, if the velocities differ, and the incidence is not normal). If the characteristic impedances are unequal, however, the incident energy is shared between waves reflected and transmitted at the boundary so as to satisfy the conditional requirements in the relationships between the particle pressures and velocities. Because velocity is a directional quantity, whereas pressure is not, the calculation requires that account should be taken of the angle of incidence at the boundary. The most useful result is that corresponding to normal incidence: in this case, the fraction, R, of the incident energy which is reflected is given by the equation

$$R = [(Z_2 - Z_1)/(Z_2 + Z_1)]^2 \tag{1.6}$$

If $Z_1 = Z_2$, $R = 0$: thus, there is no reflexion at a boundary between media of equal characteristic impedance. There is only a small reflexion at the boundary between two soft tissues, which have similar characteristic impedances. On the other hand, if $Z_2 \ll Z_1$ (for example, at the interface between soft tissue and air), then $R \simeq 1$, corresponding to almost complete reflexion.

1.1.c.   Scattering

It is important to realise that the results of calculations of refraction and reflexion conditions at a plane boundary may not apply to a similar characteristic impedance discontinuity at a rough interface or a small obstacle. The specular component of reflexion is replaced, by an amount depending upon the geometrical characteristics of the discontinuity, by components of *scattered* energy. This effect becomes important when the dimensions of the discontinuity are in the order of a wavelength or less. If the obstacle is very much less than a wavelength in size, the intensity of the wave which returns to the source (for given conditions of characteristic impedance) varies inversely as the fourth power of the wavelength. This is the situation when ultrasound of low megahertz frequency is scattered by blood. The intermediate situation, between specular reflexion and fourth-power-law scattering, is theoretically very difficult. Many of the boundaries in biological tissues are in this category, but it is only recently that experimental measurements have begun to be used to test theoretical analyses.

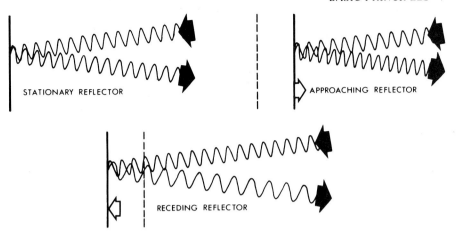

Fig. 1.3 Diagrams illustrating the Doppler shift frequency of a wave reflected by a moving surface.

Consequently, in such cases it is generally better to rely on the results of experiment in estimating reflexion conditions.

1.1.d. Doppler effect

In the situation illustrated in Fig. 1.3, the frequencies of the transmitted and the reflected waves are equal if the reflecting boundary is stationary. Movement of the reflecting boundary towards the source, however, results in a compression of the wavelength of the reflected wave, and *vice versa*. Since the velocity of propagation is constant, these changes in wavelength produce corresponding changes in frequency. The phenomenon is called the '*Doppler effect*'.

At normal incidence if f is the frequency of the incident wave, and v is the velocity of the reflecting boundary towards the source, the Doppler shift in frequency f_D which occurs in the reflected wave ($f_D = f' - f$, where f' is the received frequency) is given by

$$f_D = 2vf/c \qquad (1.7)$$

provided that $v \ll c$, as is generally the case in diagnostic applications. In these applications, it often happens that the direction of the motion of the reflecting boundary is at an angle γ with the incident wave, although the incident and reflected waves are effectively coincident. Then

$$f_D = 2v(\cos \gamma) f/c \qquad (1.8)$$

1.1.e. Power, intensity, and the decibel notation

Ultrasonic *power* may be expressed in any of several related units: one of the most useful is the *watt*. A power of 1 W is equivalent to a rate of flow of energy of 1 joule per second. The ultrasonic *intensity* is equal to the quantity of energy flowing through unit area in unit time: it may be expressed in terms of *watts per square centimetre**.

*The SI base unit is the $[\text{W m}^{-2}]$, but this involves an inconveniently large area in relation to practical situations in biomedicine. The unit $[\text{W cm}^{-2}]$ is permissible in the SI.

The intensity, I, is given by the relationship $I = \rho c v_0^2 / 2$, where v_0 is the peak particle velocity; and $v_0 = 2\pi f u_0$, where u_0 is the peak particle displacement.

The absolute value of ultrasonic intensity is an important consideration in relation to possible biological effects, and to the ability of a system to detect an ultrasonic wave in the presence of noise. It is frequently very convenient, however, to measure the *ratios* between pairs of intensities, or amplitudes, particularly if the *level* of one of these is taken as a reference for comparison with others. In this way, the need for absolute measurement is avoided, and, because ultrasonic waves are generally both generated and detected electrically, relative wave amplitudes can be expressed as ratios of voltages.

Two advantages accrue if such ratios are expressed as logarithms. Firstly, this

Table 1.2.   Power and amplitude ratios for various decibel levels.

| dB's + ve | | | dB's −ve | |
Amplitude ratio	Power ratio	dB	Amplitude ratio	Power ratio
1·000	1·000	0·0	1·000	1·000
0·989	0·977	0·1	1·012	1·022
0·977	0·955	0·2	1·023	1·047
0·944	0·891	0·5	1·059	1·122
0·891	0·794	1	1·122	1·259
0·794	0·631	2	1·259	1·585
0·708	0·501	3	1·413	1·995
0·631	0·398	4	1·585	2·512
0·562	0·316	5	1·778	3·162
0·501	0·251	6	1·995	3·981
0·447	0·200	7	2·239	5·012
0·398	0·159	8	2·512	6·310
0·355	0·126	9	2·818	7·943
0·316	0·100	10	3·162	10·000
0·282	0·0794	11	3·548	12·59
0·251	0·0631	12	3·981	15·85
0·224	0·0501	13	4·467	19·95
0·200	0·0398	14	5·012	25·12
0·178	0·0316	15	5·623	31·62
0·159	0·0251	16	6·310	39·81
0·141	0·0200	17	7·080	50·12
0·126	0·0159	18	7·943	63·10
0·112	0·0126	19	8·913	79·43
0·100	0·0100	20	10·000	100·00
0·0562	0·003 16	25	17·78	316
0·0316	0·001 00	30	31·62	1000
0·0178	0·000 32	35	56·23	3162
0·0100	0·000 10	40	100·00	10 000
0·0056	0·000 03	45	177·83	31 623
0·0032	0·000 01	50	316·23	100 000
0·001 00	10^{-6}	60	1000	10^{6}
0·000 32	10^{-7}	70	3162	10^{7}
0·000 10	10^{-8}	80	10 000	10^{8}
0·000 03	10^{-9}	90	31 623	10^{9}
0·000 01	10^{-10}	100	100 000	10^{10}

affords a simple method of expressing numbers which extend over many orders of magnitude. Secondly, the arithmetic product of two or more quantities is obtained by the addition of their logarithms (and similarly, by subtraction, in the case of division). The logarithmic unit which is most commonly used is the *decibel*, defined as follows:

$$\text{(relative level in decibels)} = 10 \log_{10}(P_2/P_1) = 20 \log_{10}(A_2/A_1), \tag{1.9}$$

where P_1 and P_2 are the two powers, and A_1 and A_2 are the corresponding wave amplitudes.

The decibel levels corresponding to a wide range of power and amplitude ratios are shown in Table 1.2. It is important to appreciate that it is meaningless to express an absolute value of any quantity in terms of decibels, unless a reference level is also stated. Thus, for example, an intensity of 40 dB below 1 W cm^{-2} is equal to $0{\cdot}0001$ W cm^{-2} (*i.e.* 10^{-4} W cm^{-2}): note that *intensities* can be compared in the same way as *powers*. Similarly, the amplitude ratio of two waves, one, 20 dB, and the other, 40 dB, below a fixed reference, is equal to 10 (*i.e.* the first wave is 20 dB greater in amplitude than the second). The *half-power distance* (the distance for half the energy to be absorbed) is almost exactly equal to the length of path traversing which the intensity falls by 3 dB.

1.1.f.   Attenuation

There are two processes by which the intensity of an ultrasonic wave may be *attenuated* during its propagation. Firstly, the wave may diverge from a parallel beam, or it may be scattered by small discontinuities in characteristic impedance, so that the ultrasonic power flows through an increased area. (Convergence of the beam results in an increase in intensity towards the focus.) Secondly, the wave may be *absorbed*, ultrasonic energy being converted into heat.

At any particular frequency, a constant fraction of the energy carried in an ultrasonic plane wave is lost by absorption in passing through a given thickness of a given material. For example, if the wave energy were to be reduced by a factor of 10 in passing through 100 mm of a certain material, then it follows that 200 mm of the material would reduce the wave energy by a factor of 100 (because the first 100 mm would absorb 90 per cent of the energy, the remaining 10 per cent being transmitted into the second 100 mm; in this, 90 per cent of the 10 per cent of the original energy would be absorbed, so that only 1 per cent would remain). In the absence of any other loss mechanism, the absorption represents the total attenuation which can be conveniently expressed in logarithmic units, such as decibels (see Section 1.1.e), because arithmetic products are obtained by the addition of logarithms. For instance, in the above example, 100 mm of material would reduce the wave energy by 10 dB, and 200 mm, by 20 dB: the *attenuation coefficient*, α, would be equal to 1 dB cm^{-1}. Hence, 120 mm would reduce the wave energy by 12 dB (and it can be seen from Table 1.2 that this corresponds to a factor of $15{\cdot}85$: it would be quite difficult to calculate this by linear arithmetic). Similarly, the half-power distance would be 30 mm.

The mechanisms by which ultrasound may be attenuated depend upon the properties of the material in which the wave is propagated. Some values for various typical materials are given in Table 1.1. In non-biological fluids, such as air and water, the attenuation coefficient is proportional to the square of the frequency; this is because absorption is due to viscosity, which itself is an aspect of friction between the particles of the fluid. In non-biological solids, absorption is mainly due to heat conduction; heat due to compression flows away so that energy is lost over the oscillation cycle, the attenuation coefficient being proportional to the frequency. In biological soft tissues, however, which are quasi-liquid, experimental measurements reveal that the attenuation coefficient is proportional to the frequency, at least over a limited frequency range. It seems that the most important contribution to absorption is due to *relaxation processes* in the protein constituents of the tissues. A relaxation process is one in which energy is first removed from the ultrasonic wave, and then returned at an appreciably later time in the wave cycle. Energy is transferred from the translational mode of motion (which is the ultrasonic wave) to other modes, such as vibration or rotation of the atoms within the molecules. Energy loss occurs when the translational motion of the ultrasonic wave is opposed by the translational motions returned to the wave from the transfer modes. The amount of energy loss depends upon the proportion of translational energy which is shared with other modes, and on the time constants of the relaxation processes. At very low frequencies, the time delay in energy transfer is negligible, and so the absorption is small. The absorption increases with increasing frequency, up to a maximum value when the shared energy is exactly opposed; above this frequency, the absorption falls because there is less time available for transfer between the energy modes. The linear relationship between the absorption coefficient and the frequency which occurs in biological soft tissues over a limited range of frequency could be due to only a few distinct relaxation processes with different time constants.

The attenuation mechanism in lung is especially complicated; the behaviour of gas-filled cavities is not fully understood in this context. Likewise, the processes which occur in bone have not been satisfactorily explained, although it seems likely that scattering may have a significant role in the diploë.

1.2. GENERATION AND DETECTION OF ULTRASONIC WAVES

1.2.a. Piezoelectricity

In diagnostic applications, ultrasound is both generated and detected by the *piezoelectric effect*. Generation and detection are processes involving conversion between electrical and mechanical energies.

Piezoelectric materials are called *'transducers'* because they provide a coupling between electrical and mechanical energies. The electric charges bound within the ionic lattice of the material are arranged in such a way that they can react with an applied electric field to produce a mechanical effect, and *vice versa*. In the undeformed state, the centre of symmetry of the positive ions coincides with that of the negative ions and, because the ionic charges are equal in magnitude but opposite in sign, there is no effective charge difference across the *crystal*. If the transducer is compressed the centres of symmetry of the ions no longer coincide, so that a charge difference appears at the electrodes. The opposite charge difference appears if the transducer is extended. The converse piezoelectric effect occurs because the application of an electric field tends to move the centres of symmetry of the ionic charges in opposite directions, causing the transducer to deform.

Although there are many natural crystals which are piezoelectric (the best-known is *quartz*), the most commonly used transducer material in ultrasonic diagnosis is the synthetic ceramic *lead zirconate titanate*. This is a solid solution which can be polarized during manufacture so that it is strongly piezoelectric. It belongs to a group of materials called *'ferroelectrics'*. In a ferroelectric material, there are many tiny electric charge domains which are preferentially orientated in a particular direction by the polarization process. These domains are asymmetrical, as illustrated in Fig. 1.4. The term *'ferroelectric'* is applied to this behaviour, because of its analogy to ferromagnetism.

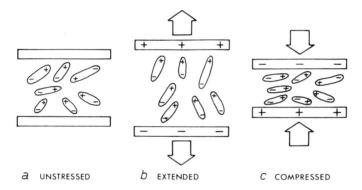

Fig. 1.4 Diagrams illustrating the interaction between force and electric charge distribution in a piezoelectric transducer of the polarised ferroelectric variety. The arrows indicate the directions of the applied stresses, and the resultant surface charges are indicated at the electrodes. The converse effect leads to deformation of the transducer in response to an applied voltage.

1.2.b.   Transducers for ultrasonic diagnosis

Narrow beams of ultrasound are almost always required in ultrasonic diagnosis. Such a beam is often generated (see Section 1.3) by a disc of piezoelectric material electrically excited by means of two electrodes, one on each parallel surface. If an alternating voltage is applied between the electrodes, the piezoelectric effect causes a synchronous variation in the thickness of the transducer.

The movements of the surfaces of the transducer radiate energy into the media which are adjacent to them; the proportion of the energy which is radiated depends upon the corresponding characteristic impedances (as discussed in Section 1.1.b). Therefore, some of the vibrational energy is, in general, reflected into the transducer at each of its surfaces: this energy travels back within the transducer. Meanwhile, if the instantaneous value of the voltage applied to the transducer is varying, a new stress situation exists (due to the piezoelectric effect) by the time that the energy reflected within the transducer arrives at the opposite surfaces. The net stress causing the transducer to deform is equal to the sum of the piezoelectric stress and the stress due to the reflected wave. If the thickness of the transducer is equal to one half a wavelength at the frequency of the electrical excitation, these stresses reinforce each other. This condition is known as 'resonance': the displacement amplitudes of the surface of the transducer are greatest when the electrical driving frequency is equal to the mechanical resonant frequency of the transducer. Similarly, the transducer has maximum sensitivity as a receiver when it is driven by ultrasound at its resonant frequency. The ultrasonic velocity in lead zirconate titanate is about $4000 \, \mathrm{m \, s^{-1}}$; and, for example, at a frequency of 1 MHz, $\lambda/2 = 2$ mm.

In some applications, it is desirable for the transducer to operate at maximum efficiency. This requires that the electrical energy should be transferred with the minimum of loss from the transducer to the load (or *vice versa*). In such a case, the transducer is backed by air, to minimise the loss in its mounting, and some improvement can be gained by *matching* the characteristic impedance of the transducer to that of the loading medium by means of a matching layer attached to the transducer, of intermediate characteristic impedance and of thickness equal to one quarter of a wavelength. A more important requirement in many diagnostic applications, however, is that the transducer should be capable of responding to energy pulses of very short duration. High efficiency transducers are generally unsatisfactory in such applications. This is because transducers of this type rely upon the oscillation reinforcement which occurs at resonance, and this is greatest when the *damping* of the transducer is minimal. The efficiency is much reduced even at frequencies which deviate only by a small amount from the resonant frequency. The *response* of the transducer, however, becomes less dependent upon the frequency as the damping is increased. Thus, the efficiency (or sensitivity) of the transducer must be reduced in order to achieve a response which is less critically dependent upon frequency.

An important property of a short-duration pulse of energy is that the energy is not confined to a single frequency. In general, the shortest pulse has the widest frequency *spectrum* of energy. Thus, in order for a transducer to respond to a short pulse of energy (which is spread over a wide frequency spectrum), it is

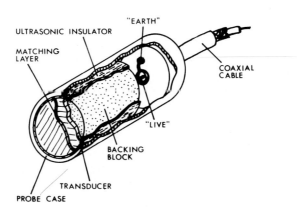

Fig. 1.5 Construction of a typical transducer probe for short pulse operation. The electrical connexions are made to thin metal electrodes bonded to the flat surfaces of the transducer. Usually, the rear electrode is *live*, and the front electrode is connected to the metal case which is *earthed*.

necessary for the transducer to be damped so that its efficiency (or sensitivity) has a wide frequency response.

Fig. 1.5 shows a typical form of construction for a probe for the generation and detection of short ultrasonic pulses. The mechanical damping is provided by a block of highly absorbent material (for example, fine particles of tungsten suspended in plastic) attached to the rear surface of the transducer. The front surface of the transducer is attached to a plastic matching layer. Ideally, this layer should be $\lambda/4$ in thickness, to achieve maximum efficiency; a compromise is necessary, however, because the wavelength is frequency-dependent, and the pulse energy extends over a wide frequency spectrum. The ultrasonic insulator (for example, rubberised cork) between the case of the probe and the transducer-backing block assembly minimises the coupling of ultrasonic energy into and from the case. Such coupling is undesirable because the case may be made of a low-loss material (for example, metal) and is likely to *ring* for some time in response to an ultrasonic transient. Ringing of the case would be detected by the transducer as an *artifact*.

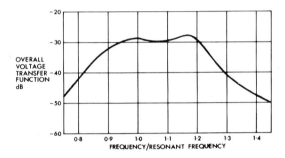

Fig. 1.6 Frequency response of a typical diagnostic ultrasonic probe.

The frequency response of a typical diagnostic ultrasonic probe is shown in Fig. 1.6. The *overall voltage transfer function* of a transducer (at any given frequency) is defined as the ratio (usually expressed in decibels) between the output and input voltages across the transducer, when the transmitted ultrasonic energy is reflected back to the probe without loss. In practice, a perfect reflector is difficult to construct, and a flat reflector of known reflectivity is used, appropriate corrections being made to the measurements of transfer function.

The pulse response of the same probe is shown in Fig. 1.7. The pulse shape can be specified in terms of its *zero-crossing frequency,* and *duration* between specified *threshold* levels below the *peak amplitude*. These are important quantities in the estimation of the *resolution* of a pulse-echo diagnostic system (see Section 2.1.c).

1.3. THE ULTRASONIC FIELD

1.3.a.   Steady state conditions

The '*ultrasonic field*' of a transducer is the term used to describe the spatial distribution of its radiated energy. By reciprocity, this is identical to the sensitivity distribution of the transducer when acting as a receiver.

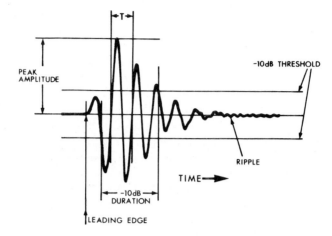

Fig. 1.7 Pulse response of a typical diagnostic ultrasonic probe. The zero-crossing frequency is equal to $1/T$. The ripple which follows the pulse is due to *ringing* of the probe case, and to radial-mode resonance of the transducer.

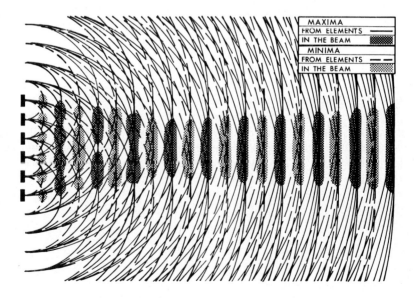

Fig. 1.8 Diagram illustrating the formation of an ultrasonic beam by a six-element linear array.

The analysis of the ultrasonic field is based on the application of *Huygen's construction,* in which the surface of the transducer is considered to be an array of separate elements each radiating spherical waves in the forward direction. The elements move in synchrony with equal amplitudes (*i.e.* a disc transducer is considered to be a piston the surface of which vibrates cophasally at constant amplitude). This is known as a *'steady state'* condition. The method of analysis is illustrated in Fig. 1.8 by a simple example, in which the source consists of a six-element linear array. The waves *interfere* constructively to reinforce each other along the lines which touch the spherical waves due to every element. In other places, there is a tendency for maxima and minima to coincide, so that destructive interference occurs, and there is little net disturbance. Consequently, the ultrasonic field is concentrated within a *beam,* and this becomes more uniform with increasing distance from the array.

It is relatively easy to apply Huygen's construction to the analysis of one dimension of the ultrasonic field of a linear array. The situation is much more complicated, however, if the source is in the form of, for example, a circular piston. The problem is one of three-dimensional geometry: the theoretical field for such a source is shown diagrammatically in Fig. 1.9. Moving along the central axis of the beam towards the source, the intensity increases until a maximum is reached at a distance x'_{max} from the source given by

$$x'_{max} = r^2/\lambda \qquad (1.10)$$

where r is the radius of the source and $r^2 \gg \lambda^2$ (as is usually the case in ultrasonic diagnosis). Increasingly closely spaced axial maxima and minima occur towards the source. At successive axial maxima and minima, starting at x'_{max} and moving towards the source, there are one, two, three, *etc.*, principal maxima across the beam diameter. Thus, the beam contains two distinct regions. The region between the source and the last axial maximum (at x'_{max}) is known as the *'near field'* (or Frésnel zone); the region beyond this is the *'far field'* (or Fraunhofer

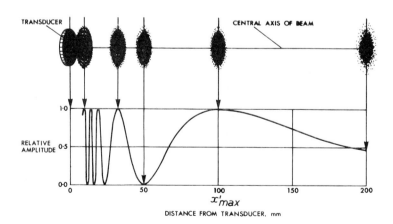

Fig. 1.9 The ultrasonic field. This example shows the distribution for a 1·5 MHz transducer of radius
$r = 10$ mm. The ultrasonic beam normal to the central axis is circular in section, and the
elliptical diagrams represent such sections, in the planes indicated on the graph. The graph
shows the variation in the central axial amplitude with distance from the transducer.

zone). The beam is roughly cylindrical in the near field. Deep in the far field, the beam diverges at angles $\pm\theta$ about the central axis, given by

$$\sin\theta = 0.61\lambda/r \qquad (1.11)$$

Thus, the shape of the ultrasonic field depends upon the diameter of the transducer and the wavelength of the ultrasound. For example, a transducer of 20 mm diameter operating at 1·5 MHz in water has a near field length of 100 mm and a half-angle of divergence of 3·5° in the far field. The length of the near field increases with increasing diameter of the transducer and increasing frequency of the ultrasound (because $\lambda = c/f$); but the divergence in the far field decreases with increasing diameter and increasing frequency.

1.3.b. Transient conditions
In the steady state, the shape of the ultrasonic field is determined by interference between contributions from the entire surface of the source. If a short-duration pulse of ultrasound is involved, however, all the contributions which combine together to form the field in the steady state may not be present at any particular point in space during the passage of the transient. This is because, in general, the surface of the source is not equidistant from the point (except at the focus of a curved transducer). Consequently, the field shape changes with time. In the far field, steady state conditions apply within about half a cycle of the arrival of the transient; but in the near field, the transition between transient and steady state conditions may occupy from 3 to 6 half-cycles. The matter is rather complicated, and in any event it has little practical importance in ultrasonic diagnosis, because experimental measurements of beam shape can be made under transient conditions if this is appropriate.

1.3.c. Focused fields
In most diagnostic applications, it is desirable for the ultrasonic beamwidth to be minimal. In the case of a plane disc transducer, the shape of the field depends upon its diameter, and the frequency of the ultrasound (as discussed in Section 1.3.a). To some extent, these factors are determined by the nature of the diagnostic investigation. Thus, the penetration is reduced with increasing

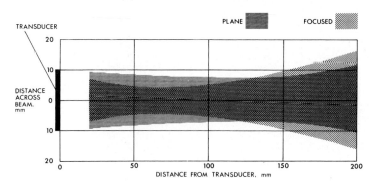

Fig. 1.10 The effect of focusing on the beam width. This example shows the typical effective beamwidths for a 1·5 MHz transducer of radius $r = 10$ mm. The focused transducer has a radius of curvature of 100 mm.

frequency (because of the corresponding increase in attenuation: the frequency is generally chosen to be as high as possible within this limitation). At any given frequency, the width of the ultrasonic beam in the near field is reduced by reducing the diameter of the transducer, but this also reduces the length of the near field and increases the divergence in the far field. Focusing can give an improvement, however, in the beamwidth over a limited part of the field. Focusing can be achieved by lenses, or by mirrors, or by appropriately shaped transducers. An example of the improvement in the beamwidth which can be obtained by this method is shown in Fig. 1.10.

1.3.d. Arrays

A probe containing several separate transducer elements, each electrically and acoustically isolated, is called an 'array'. There are two distinct types of array. In one type, each element in the array is operated independently of the others, so that the shape of the beam which it produces can be predicted on the basis of the treatment in the earlier part of this Section. In the other type of array, two or more elements are operated together to produce a beam which depends upon the configurations of all the transducers involved, and also on the characteristics of their excitation signals and receiver signal processing. If an adequate number of elements of sufficiently small size is involved, Huygen's construction may be used to calculate the shape of the ultrasonic field.

Arrays have their chief application in rapid scanning systems (see Section 2.1.e). They are also used to generate a swept focus which overcomes the depth-of-focus limitation of static systems.

FOR FURTHER READING

WELLS, P.N.T. (1977). *Biomedical Ultrasonics*. London and New York: Academic Press.

2. Diagnostic methods

P.N.T. WELLS

Ultrasonic diagnosis is based, with very few exceptions, upon the reflexion of ultrasonic waves which occurs at the boundaries between different tissues within the body. A fraction of the incident ultrasonic energy is reflected if there is a change in characteristic impedance at such a boundary. Although the echoes which correspond to soft tissue boundaries have very small amplitudes,* they can be detected by a sensitive receiver. The energy which is not reflected travels beyond the boundary, and may be reflected at deeper boundaries. The maximum penetration is limited by the attenuation of the ultrasound in passing through the tissues.

Ultrasound is almost completely reflected at boundaries with gas. This prevents examination through gas, and is a serious restriction in investigations of and through gas-containing structures. In addition, it is necessary to exclude air from between the transducer and the patient: this is done by means of a liquid coupling medium.

The attenuation rate and the propagation velocity are both much higher in bone than in soft tissues. Consequently, examinations through bone are difficult, and they are only really satisfactory in a few specific applications.

2.1 PULSE-ECHO METHODS

An ultrasonic pulse is reflected when it strikes the boundary between two media of differing characteristic impedance, and the time delay which occurs between the transmission of the pulse and the reception of its echo depends upon the propagation velocity and the path length. Range-measuring systems based on this principle are widely applied in medical diagnostics. The propagation velocities are similar in different soft tissues, and any error introduced by assuming a constant relationship between time and distance can usually be neglected. At a velocity of 1500 m s^{-1}, ultrasound travels 10 mm in about 6.7 μs.

2.1.a.   The A-scope

The basis of the pulse-echo method is illustrated in Fig. 2.1. The diagrams show how an ultrasonic pulse may be used to measure the depth of an echo-producing boundary. If the process is repeated sufficiently rapidly (at a rate greater than about 20 times per second), the persistence of vision of the observer gives the impression of a steady trace on the display. In soft tissues, the ultrasonic echoes are delayed in time from the transmission pulse by about 13.3 μs for each

*For example, substitution of the appropriate values in Equation 1.6 (Section 1.1.b) shows that, at a flat interface between kidney and fat, about 0.6 per cent of the incident energy is reflected.

centimetre of penetration, during which time the ultrasonic pulse travels along a total go-and-return path length of 20 mm.

The kind of display illustrated in Fig. 2.1. is called an 'A-scan'. (This term, like several others used in ultrasonics, is the same as that which describes the equivalent display in radar.) The method can be extended to the examination of many interfaces lying along the ultrasonic path.

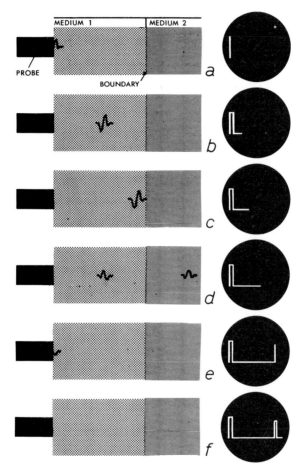

Fig. 2.1 Basic principles of the pulse-echo system. (a) The probe emits a short-duration ultrasonic pulse into medium 1, and simultaneously the spot on the cathode ray tube display begins to move at constant velocity from left to right. The vertical deflexion plates of the cathode ray tube are connected to the output from an amplifier, the input of which is derived from the ultrasonic probe. The spot is deflected vertically at the instant that the ultrasonic pulse is emitted, because the exciting voltage is also applied to the amplifier. (b) The ultrasonic pulse travels along a narrow beam at constant velocity through medium 1, and the spot traces a horizontal line on the display. (c) The ultrasonic pulse reaches the boundary between media 1 and 2. (d) If there is a characteristic impedance discontinuity at the boundary, some of the ultrasonic energy is reflected back into medium 1. (e) The reflected wave reaches the probe, and generates a voltage which produces a second deflexion on the display. (f) The distance between the two deflexions on the display is proportional to the distance between the probe and the boundary between the two media.

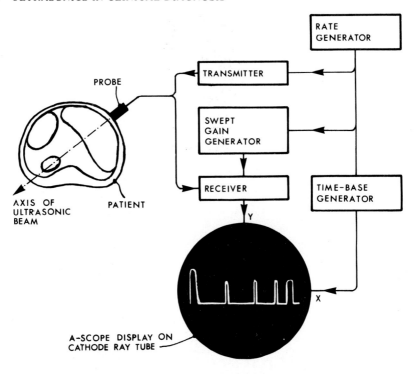

Fig. 2.2 Basic elements of the A-scope system. The output from the receiver is connected to the vertical (Y) deflexion plates of the cathode ray tube, and that from the time-base generator, to the horizontal (X) plates. (Courtesy: the Editor, *Journal of the Royal College of Physicians.*)

The basic elements of an A-scope system are shown in the block diagram in Fig. 2.2. The rate generator simultaneously triggers the transmitter, the swept gain generator, and the time-base generator. The voltages which appear at the probe are amplified by the receiver, and applied to the vertical deflexion plates of the cathode ray tube. The output from the time-base generator is applied to the horizontal deflexion plates.

A substantial improvement in the usefulness of the displayed information is obtained if the echo signals from deeper structures are amplified more than those which originate closer to the probe. This function is performed by the swept gain generator, which is arranged to increase the gain of the receiver with time at an appropriate rate. Ideally, swept gain should lead to similar registrations of similar surfaces, irrespective of their distances from the probe. In practice, however, accurate swept gain is difficult to achieve, for two main reasons. Firstly, there is a variation in the attenuation rates of different tissues. Secondly, the energy in the ultrasonic pulse is distributed over quite a wide frequency spectrum, and the higher frequency components of the pulse are increasingly attenuated with increasing penetration (the attenuation coefficients in soft tissues are approximately proportional to the frequency).

In certain circumstances, diagnostic information may be obtained by studying the amplitudes of the displayed echoes. Such investigations are often made easier if swept gain is applied to the system: it is essential in gray-scale scanning, to obtain the potential advantages of the method (see Section 2.1.e). It is important to remember that an extensive smooth surface gives rise to specular reflexion, and so the amplitude of the echo received from such a surface is very directionally dependent; but the echo from a small discontinuity, although smaller in amplitude, is less markedly directional.

Although in a few systems there is a linear relationship between the input and output signals of the receiver, it is more usual for some form of *signal processing* to be used. Thus, the signal is generally *demodulated* so that the output is a unidirectional representation of the alternating voltage which occurs at the probe. In addition, the *dynamic range* of the input signals may be compressed, so that a wide variation in amplitude at the input produces a smaller variation at the output: this may be achieved by an amplifier with a logarithmic characteristic.

2.1.b. Operation of the A-scope
A-scope systems are normally fitted with a number of manually operated controls. There is considerable variation in this respect between different instruments. A brief description of the more important of their functions is given here.

(i) *Rate generator*
The *repetition rate* of the system may be adjustable. A higher repetition rate gives a brighter display, but restricts the maximum penetration (because the interval between the ultrasonic pulses becomes closer to the time during which echoes are being received), and increases the possibility of biological hazard.

(ii) *Transmitter*
A variable *attenuator* may be fitted to control the amplitude of the transmitted ultrasonic pulse. This has the effect of controlling the overall sensitivity of the system.

(iii) *Swept gain generator*
The characteristics of the swept gain function, such as its *timing* and its *rate,* may be adjustable. It may be possible to display simultaneously the A-scan and the swept gain function, so that the effect of the latter may be more easily appreciated.

(iv) *Receiver*
This may be fitted with a variable *gain* control, to adjust the sensitivity of the system (in view of the possibility of biological hazard, this is a less desirable method of sensitivity control than is provided by the transmitter attenuator in (ii) above), and a variable *suppression* control, to reject small echoes from the display. In most systems, the demodulated signal is displayed; but in some instruments, it is possible for the undemodulated signal to be displayed. In addition, the operating *frequency* may be adjustable, often within preset limits about a specified centre frequency.

(v) *Time-base generator*
The *velocity* of the time-base may be adjustable. A *time-marker* circuit is

sometimes included: this generates time-markers on the display at positions corresponding to known intervals of distance in soft tissues.

(vi) *Display*

This may have the usual controls for the adjustments of *focus, brightness* and *astigmatism.* It may be possible to *invert* the trace, and to *shift* it both horizontally and vertically.

2.1.c.   Multiple reflexion artifacts

A serious limitation of the pulse-echo method is due to the *multiple reflexions,* or reverberations, that the ultrasonic pulse may suffer during its propagation. For example, in Fig. 2.1 the pulse which returns to the probe from the boundary between the two media, and which causes the corresponding deflexion of the spot, is not completely attenuated within the probe. This is because there is a characteristic impedance discontinuity at the probe surface, and quite a large proportion of the echo energy is reflected back into the first medium, This reflected pulse behaves as if it were a second transmitted pulse, of smaller amplitude than the first, delayed in time by an interval equal to the delay in the return of the first echo. Consequently, a second echo returns from the boundary

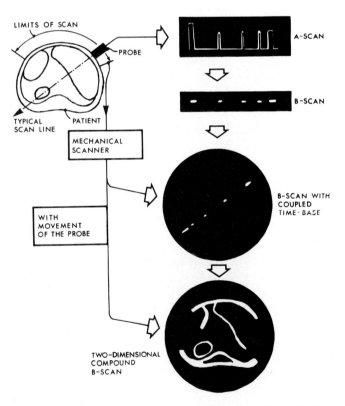

Fig. 2.3 Diagrams illustrating the relationship between the A-scan and B-scan displays, and the basic principles of two-dimensional ultrasonic scanning. (Courtesy: the Editor, *Journal of the Royal College of Physicians.*)

between the first and second media, and this produces a registration on the display at a position corresponding to twice the range of the boundary. Similarly, third and subsequent reverberation *artifacts* appear, until the ultrasonic pulse becomes too small to be detected.

Multiple reflexions causing artifacts are sometimes quite easily recognised by the regularity of their spacings. Those due to gas and bone are a fundamental limitation in ultrasonic diagnostics.

2.1.d.   The B-scope

The information obtained with a pulse-echo system is a combination of range and amplitude data which can often be conveniently presented as an A-scan. The same information, however, may alternatively be displayed on a brightness-modulated time-base, in such a way that the brightness increases with the echo amplitude, as shown in Fig. 2.3. This type of display is called a *'B-scan'*. The B-scope is the basis of the two-dimensional scanner (see Section 2.1.e) and the most common types of time-position recorder (see Section 2.1.i).

2.1.e.   The two-dimensional B-scope

It is possible to mount the ultrasonic probe on a mechanical scanner which allows movements in two dimensions, and which links (either electrically or mechanically) the direction and position of a B-scope time-base on a cathode ray tube to those of the ultrasonic beam within the patient. Then, by continuously recording the display whilst the probe is moved around the patient, a cross-sectional picture in the plane of the scan (a *tomograph*) is constructed in two dimensions. The process is illustrated in Fig. 2.3. The continuous recording process may be either photographic (often using 'Polaroid'* film, which allows the finished scan to be viewed with the minimum of delay) or electronic. Electronic recording may be either by direct view storage tube (bistable or transmission control), or, for gray scale, by scan converter with television monitor.

Until recently, ultrasonic two-dimensional scanners were generally designed chiefly to produce tissue *'maps'*, in which the emphasis was on the display of organ boundaries. The 'best' scans were considered to be those in which the anatomy was depicted by thin white lines on a black background. For this purpose, the *dynamic range* of the display was unimportant.

The dynamic range of the display is a measure of its ability to represent input amplitude variation in terms of spot brightness. It may be expressed as the decibel ratio between the minimum input amplitude at which a registration is just visible on the display, and the maximum input amplitude above which there is no further visible increase in brightness. A second, and equally important, consideration is the number of separate shades of brightness which may be identified on the display over its dynamic range. This depends on a number of factors, including both the technical properties of the display, and the psychophysics of the observer. Some general principles are illustrated in Fig. 2.4.

Nowadays, there is much emphasis on gray scale capability in two-dimensional scanning. Unlike the bistable or low dynamic range display which

*Registered Trademark of Polaroid Corporation, Cambridge, MA 02139, USA.

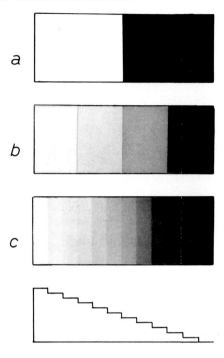

Fig. 2.4 Display dynamic range and gray scale capability. The graph at the bottom of the diagram represents the input amplitude. (*a*) This is a *bistable* display, in which there is a threshold input level above which the display is fully white, and below which it is fully black. (*b*) In this display, there are two discernible brightnesses between white and black, and the *gray scale* has 4 levels. (*c*) This gray scale has 12 discernible levels.

was used for tissue mapping, the gray scale display allows deductions to be made from the scan concerning quite subtle characteristics of the echo amplitudes arising from within organs and structures.

The angles of incidence and reflexion of an ultrasonic beam are equal at a flat surface. The maximum echo amplitude is detected at normal incidence, since only then does the echo return directly to the transducer. Consequently, in conventional tissue-mapping applications at least, an improved image (a *compound B-scan*) is obtained if the probe is oscillated as it is moved around the patient, because this increases the likelihood of the occurrence of normal incidence with specular reflectors. Complete information cannot be obtained in this way, however, if the surface being examined is not normal to the plane of the scan, nor is it usually possible to scan through a complete circle.

There are many different designs of two-dimensional ultrasonic scanner. They can be conveniently divided into two main groups, according to whether the transducer scans the patient through an intervening water bath, or by direct contact with the patient's skin. *Water bath* scanners have the advantages that the movements of the probe may be automatic, and that the patient may be scanned in the far field of the ultrasonic beam. Also, the patient may be examined without any local disturbance of body structures being caused by the movement of the probe. On the other hand, there may be considerable difficulty in achieving a satisfactory coupling between the patient and the water (unless immersion is possible), because air is likely to be trapped between the flexible membrane, which forms the wall of the water tank, and the patient's skin. This difficulty restricts the areas of the body which can be examined by the method. *Contact* scanners are versatile in this respect, although they are unsuitable for examining small organs (like the eye), or soft structures where information is required from close to the skin (such as the breast). Consequently, this kind of scanner is widely used in abdominal investigations; the probe is generally moved by hand, and the ultrasonic coupling is provided by a film of oil smeared on the patient's skin. The coupling is satisfactory, provided that the angle through which the probe is oscillated to 'compound' the scan is not made too great.

The various types of commercially available conventional scanners in common use and based on single-element transducers are illustrated in Fig. 2.5. Another group of scanners is capable of real-time visualization, either by fast

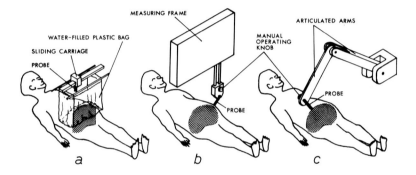

Fig. 2.5 The various types of commercially available two-dimensional B-scanner in common use, based on single-element transducers. The stippled areas indicate the scan planes. (*a*) A water-bath scanner with a linear scan pattern. (*b*) A manually-operated scanner with a rectilinear measuring frame. (*c*) A manually-operated contact scanner with articulated arms working in polar coordinates. See Appendix (at end of book) for further details of these systems.

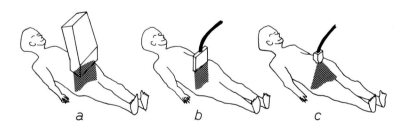

Fig. 2.6 Various types of two-dimensional real-time scanners. The stippled areas indicate the scan planes. (*a*) A water-bath scanner with a rotating transducer assembly mounted at the focus of a parabolic mirror: this produces a linear scan pattern. (*b*) A linear array of transducers, operated sequentially in groups: this produces a linear scan pattern. (*c*) A linear transducer array: the phasing across the array is controlled electronically to produce a sector scan. See Appendix (at end of book) for further details of these systems.

mechanical operation of a single element transducer, or by means of a transducer array. Some examples of these scanners are illustrated in Fig. 2.6.

2.1.f.   Resolution in pulse-echo systems

The *resolution* of a pulse-echo system is defined as the reciprocal of the distance which appears on the display to be occupied by a small reflector in the ultrasonic field. As in the definitions of display dynamic range and gray scale (see Section 2.1.e), considerations of the psychophysics of vision are involved in this definition.

Two different resolutions are of importance: these are the *lateral resolution*, which describes the resolution along the beam diameter normal to the axis, and the *range resolution*, which is the resolution along the axis.

The range resolution depends upon the shape of the ultrasonic echo, and the characteristics of the receiver. The waveform of a typical echo pulse at the output from the transducer is shown in Fig. 1.7. Given such an echo, the resolution corresponds to the time interval during which the echo amplitude is large enough to produce a registration on the display. Some systems respond only to the leading edge of the echo, and so the 'resolution' seems to be better than pulse length considerations would indicate: such a display is said to be *differentiated*.

The lateral resolution depends upon the effective width of the ultrasonic beam and the characteristics of the receiver. For example, the beam shape of a typical probe is shown in Fig. 2.7. At any given range, the resolution corresponds to the width of the beam from within which the echo amplitude from a point reflector is large enough to produce a registration on the display.

These definitions neglect the complication of gray scale in discussing resolution. It may be more meaningful to define the resolution as the reciprocal of the minimum distance between two point objects in the ultrasonic field, which produces separable registrations on the display. Whilst this is a useful concept, it does involve two difficulties. The first is the psychophysical problem of defining perceptible brightness differences. The second is a physical problem which arises because the echoes from adjacent targets may interfere, destructively or constructively according to their phase relationship.

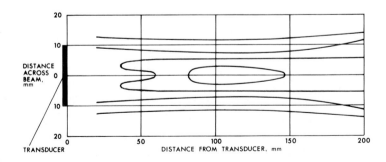

Fig. 2.7   Typical ultrasonic beam distribution. This example shows *iso-echo amplitude lines* (lines joining points at which a small spherical target in water gives echoes of equal amplitude) for a 1·5 MHz transducer of radius 10 mm, in the plane of the central axis of the beam. Spacing between adjacent lines = 10 dB.

Elementary considerations indicate that the resolution should improve with increasing frequency. The attenuation coefficient of soft tissues increases with frequency, however, and this leads to a reduction in the maximum penetration (because there is a limitation to the maximum amplification of the receiver). In addition, the errors in the swept gain compensation increase as the range of the swept gain control is increased to compensate for the greater attenuation at higher frequencies. These errors lead to a deterioration in the resolution which may offset any theoretical advantage of operating at a higher frequency. Optimum results are obtained in abdominal and neurological investigations at frequencies of 1−2 MHz, in cardiovascular work at 2−5 MHz, and in ophthalmology at 8−20 MHz. It is helpful to consider the wavelength to be the factor which controls the dimensions of the ultrasonic field. In most applications, a transducer diameter of 20λ, and a penetration of 200λ, give satisfactory results. As mentioned in Section 1.3.c, some improvement in lateral resolution can be obtained by focusing the beam.

2.1.g.   Performance of the two-dimensional B-scope

The diagnostic value of the two-dimensional pictures obtained with a B-scope scanner depends upon many factors. Elementary precautions include the necessity to ensure good ultrasonic coupling between the probe and the patient, and to maintain a reasonable degree of consistency in the movement of the probe. The appearance of the scan is also controlled by the performance of the signal processing circuits, which are similar to those of the A-scope (Sections 2.1.a and 2.1.b) with the addition of arrangements for the brightness-modulation of the display. In general, the quality of the pictures as a map of tissue boundaries is improved if its information content is increased by operating with the highest possible repetition rate, and by scanning for the longest possible time for which the patient can remain still.

The requirement of consistency in the scanning pattern is particularly important if it is desired to obtain information about echo amplitude from the brightness of the image. Photographic recording is inherently accompanied by integration; the same applies to the transmission control storage tube, although its dynamic range is rather small. Consequently the brightness of the image depends not only upon the amplitude of the echo, but also upon the scanning time. To a large extent this difficulty is overcome by a scan converter operated in the *equilibrium writing mode.* In this mode, the stored image corresponds to the highest echo amplitude received from each scanned element, to a first approximation independent of the scanning time.

In addition to considerations of resolution (Section 2.1.f), the scan quality depends upon the accuracy of the *registration* of the positions of echo-producing structures on the display. The accuracy of the registration describes how nearly a point reflector in the scan plane is represented as a single point on the display when examined by the probe from several different positions. Most systems, in which the scan is not compounded, cannot be tested in this way (because a point reflector can only be detected from one position of the probe); but poor registration can spoil a compound scan to such an extent that it is diagnostically valueless. Good registration depends upon a rigid scanning mechanism, a uniform ultrasonic beam, and accurate tracking in the linkages between the position and direction of the ultrasonic beam and those of the time-base. Fundamental limitations in the accuracy of tracking are due to errors in range due to variation in the propagation velocities in different tissues, and in azimuth due to refraction and variations in attenuation across the beam.

2.1.h. The C-scope

The *C-scope* is a brightness-modulated display of a scan plane in which deflexion along one axis corresponds to the angular position (the *azimuth*) of the echo-producing structure, and that along the other axis, to the corresponding distance from a reference datum (the *elevation*). The display is somewhat similar to a conventional x-ray picture, because it is in the form of a plan 'view'; but unlike the x-ray, the depth and thickness of the section can be controlled by electronic time-gating of the echo signals. The method is not much used in clinical diagnostics, although it is the most convenient display in the investigation of atrial septal defects using an intracardiac probe mounted at the tip of a catheter.

2.1.i. Time-position recording

Pulse-echo information from moving structures can be recorded to generate time-position waveforms. The simplest technique is to photograph a B-scan display with a camera in which the film is moving at constant velocity in a direction at right angles to the ultrasonic time-base. In modern instruments, the recording is made in this way by means of a fibre-optic cathode ray tube with self-

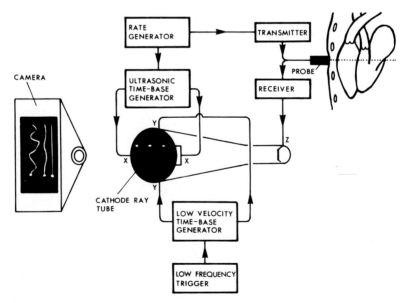

Fig. 2.8 Photographic system for time-position recording. The output from the receiver is arranged to brightness (Z) modulate the display, which is a B-scope with the output from the ultrasonic time-base applied to the horizontal (X) deflexion plates of the cathode ray tube. The vertical (Y) deflexion plates are connected to the output from a low velocity time-base generator (sweep time approximately 3 s), which may be triggered repetitively, or by a manual single-shot control.

processing paper sensitive to ultraviolet radiation. Alternatively, as shown in Fig. 2.8, the B-scan may be moved across the display at constant velocity by a second, relatively slow-speed time-base generator (connected to the appropriate pair of deflexion plates in the cathode ray tube), the recording being made either by a still camera, or on an electronic storage tube.

These methods permit the simultaneous recording of the movements of all the structures lying in the ultrasonic beam. In some circumstances, however, such as in the assessment of mitral valve function, adequate diagnostic information can be obtained by studying the movement of only one structure (for example, the anterior cusp of the mitral valve) lying in the ultrasonic beam. If the amplitude of the echo of interest is always the largest of any that occur on that part of the time-base along which it oscillates, it is possible to arrange for the echo to trigger a *time-to-voltage analogue converter*. The echo is selected electronically by means of a gate which is closed to those echoes (and the transmission pulse) which always occur before the arrival of the echo of interest. The brief interval of time (in the order of micro-seconds) between the opening of the gate, and the arrival of the echo, is converted to a voltage the amplitude of which is proportional to the time interval. This voltage analogue signal may be maintained for a relatively long time (limited by the repetition rate of the system), and this allows the motion of the echo-producing structure to be displayed on paper by means of a pen recorder. This is not possible by direct recording of the ultrasonic signals, because the times involved are too short for a pen recorder to be able to respond. The output from the analogue converter may be displayed as a continuous trace. It was this method of recording which was used for the early development of echocardiography in the 1960s, but it has largely fallen into disuse with the advent of the fibre-optic ultraviolet recorder.

2.2 DOPPLER METHODS

Ultrasonic Doppler methods are nowadays both widely used and of established value in the study of moving structures in clinical diagnosis. In most applications, the Doppler shift in frequency of a continuous wave ultrasonic beam reflected from a moving structure is used to provide information about the velocity of the structure, either for interpretation by ear, or for analysis by instrument.

The same restrictions and limitations (such as the necessity to maintain good ultrasonic coupling, and the inability to operate successfully through gas) which apply to ultrasonic pulse-echo methods, also apply to ultrasonic Doppler methods.

The choice of the ultrasonic frequency depends upon the clinical application. A compromise is necessary between the penetration, the variation of Doppler shift frequency for a given variation in target velocity, the sensitivity to small reflectors and the size and shape of the ultrasonic field. In both obstetrics and cardiology, the frequency is generally 2–3 MHz, but, in blood flow studies, it may be as high as 10 MHz.

The relationship between ultrasonic frequency, Doppler shift frequency, reflector velocity and angulation, is given by Equation 1.8 (Section 1.1d). For example, in the case where no correction for angulation is required (*i.e.* cos γ = 1), a 2 MHz ultrasonic beam is shifted in frequency by about 260 Hz after reflexion from a surface moving at a velocity of 100 mm s^{-1}. For practical purposes, the Doppler shift frequency may be taken to be proportional both to the ultrasonic frequency and to the reflector velocity.

2.2.a.   Continuous wave Doppler systems

A block diagram of a continuous wave ultrasonic Doppler frequency shift detector is shown in Fig. 2.9. The transmitter operates continuously, providing

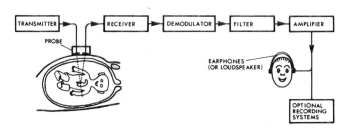

Fig. 2.9 Basic elements of the continuous-wave ultrasonic Doppler frequency shift detector.

an output of constant amplitude and frequency. The ultrasonic probe contains separate transmitting and receiving transducers. These are necessary because it is important to minimize the direct transfer of energy from the transmitter to the receiver, in order to avoid overloading the receiver amplifier. The output from the receiver consists of a mixture of signals, some of a frequency equal to that of the transmitter (these are due to reflexions from stationary structures in the ultrasonic field, and electrical leakage), and some of frequencies shifted by the Doppler effect (these are due to reflexions from moving structures). These signals are *mixed* in the demodulator, the output from which contains the difference frequencies between the transmitted ultrasonic wave and the Doppler shifted received waves. The output from the demodulator is filtered to remove signals of unwanted frequencies, and the remaining Doppler shifted signals are further amplified.

In clinical applications, the Doppler shifted signals generally do not consist of a single frequency, but they extend over a frequency spectrum. This is because the system simultaneously detects the movements of several different structures: for example, blood cells move at differing velocities in a blood vessel according to the flow profile. For this reason, measurements of Doppler shift signals made by ratemeters (which can only indicate some kind of frequency average) need to be interpreted with caution. The ear is extraordinarily good at recognising sound patterns in complex spectra, and it is often most convenient, in clinical practice, simply to listen to the Doppler shift signals. Used in this way, the Doppler system can be considered to be an active stethoscope of great sensitivity and excellent directivity. In some applications, such as in studies of blood flow, additional information can be obtained by frequency analysis of the Doppler shifted signals. (A frequency spectrum analyser is an instrument which generates a chart in which time and frequency are plotted on orthogonal axes, and the corresponding sound intensity is represented according to the density of the recording.)

2.2.b. Directionally sensitive Doppler systems

Simple continuous wave Doppler systems of the type described in Section 2.2.a do not provide information concerning the *direction* of movement of a reflector: they only indicate its *velocity,* which may be either towards or away from the probe. The directional information is defined by the arithmetic sign of f_D as given by Equations 1.7 and 1.8 (Section 1.1.d), but this is rather difficult to determine because $f_D \ll f$. There are two chief ways in which this directional information may be obtained. The first method, which is the method most commonly used in commercial instruments, simply indicates *'forward'* or *'reverse'* flow: it is clearly misleading when both forward and reverse flows exist simultaneously! The second method really depends on frequency spectrum analysis, and it is capable of displaying a spectrum of velocities, simultaneously both forward and reverse.

2.2.c. Range-gated Doppler systems

Continuous wave Doppler systems do not provide information concerning the distances from the probe to the moving structures which give rise to the shifted frequencies. It is possible, however, to separate the Doppler signals by a range-gating technique in which the frequencies of the echoes selected from a sample of distance lying between chosen limits are compared with that of a continuously running oscillator which itself gated to provide the transmitted pulse. Several systems capable of extracting this information from the Doppler signals have been devised (including some which also provide directional information), but the method is not yet widely used.

2.2.d. Two-dimensional Doppler scanning

The Doppler shifted signals from flowing blood are sufficiently characteristic to allow them to be identified by electronic logic circuitry. This ability is exploited in a two-dimensional scanner designed to map out blood vessels. The position of the Doppler probe in space in a two-dimensional plane is measured by means of resolvers mounted on a scanning frame, and this information is used to control the horizontal and vertical deflexion circuits of a cathode ray tube display. The output from the Doppler detector controls the brightness of the display. The probe is scanned regularly over the entire surface of skin beneath which it is desired to map the blood vessels, and only when the ultrasonic beam passes through moving blood does a registration appear on the display. Arterial and venous blood are distinguished by their different flow directions. The simpler two-dimensional Doppler scanners use continuous waves, but the more complicated scanners use range-finding Dopplers and are in principle capable of producing cross-sectional images of blood vessels.

2.3. OTHER METHODS

2.3.a. Transmission imaging

The earliest attempts to use ultrasound in medical diagnostics were based on the expectation that it would be possible to distinguish tissues according to their differing ultrasonic attenuations, by analogy with conventional x-radiography. These attempts failed, because of the large differences between the attenuation of soft tissues and bone or gas. From time to time, fresh work is done aimed at overcoming these difficulties. In principle, there are two types of image converter which have been tried.

The ultrasonic image camera employs a piezoelectric transducer on which an ultrasonic pattern is arranged to fall, after transmission through the object under investigation. The ultrasonic field causes a corresponding electrical charge pattern to appear on the opposite side of the transducer, and this pattern is scanned by an electron beam (in a vacuum tube). Thus, electrical signals are generated which allow an image of the object to be presented on a television-type display.

The second type of image converter uses an array of transducers which is arranged to scan the transmitted ultrasonic field. One-dimensional arrays require mechanical scanning, but two-dimensional arrays can be scanned electrically.

No significant application for any of these methods has yet been found in connexion with the solution of clinical diagnostic problems.

2.3.b.   Ultrasonic holography

Ultrasonic holography is a two-stage process of imaging analogous to optical holography. The object to be visualized is uniformly irradiated with ultrasound, and the reflected waves are sampled over a large area. The hologram is generated by recording the sum of the reflected waves and a reference wave, which may be either ultrasonic or electronic. A three-dimensional image of the original object is reconstructed when the hologram is illuminated by coherent light, such as that from a laser.

A great deal of effort has been devoted to testing the possibility of using ultrasonic holography in clinical diagnosis. The results have been very disappointing, and it is easy to understand some of the physical reasons for this. They include poor signal-to-noise ratio, degradation of phase coherence, specular reflectors, and reconstruction distortion.

FOR FURTHER READING

WELLS, P.N.T. (1977). *Biomedical Ultrasonics.* London and New York: Academic Press.

PART II   DIAGNOSTIC APPLICATIONS

3. Ultrasonic investigation of the brain

D.N. WHITE

3.1. MIDLINE ECHOENCEPHALOGRAPHY

Midline echoencephalography measures, by means of an ultrasonic pulse-echo technique (see Chapter 2), the range of the structures that lie in the cerebral median sagittal plane from the overlying scalp surface. Any significant difference in the ranges measured from either side of the head suggests that the cerebral midline structures have been displaced from the median sagittal plane by some deforming cerebral disorder. An expanding lesion such as a brain tumour or blood clot in one hemisphere displaces the midline structures towards the opposite side while an atrophic lesion, such as an old injury or thrombosis, draws the cerebral midline towards the affected side.

This is the principle of midline echoencephalography. It sounds remarkably simple. In practice it is by no means simple and the laws of acoustics coupled with the acoustic properties of the skull impose a number of severe restrictions upon the technique.

Interfaces in the soft tissues of the body vary in their reflecting characteristics. Small discontinuities, approximating to cells in size, scatter energy diffusely from their surfaces so that it is both of low intensity and attenuates rapidly at increasing distances. Large planar interfaces, such as the surfaces of organs, specularly reflect collimated energy in a collimated fashion so that these echoes are of much higher intensity and attenuate much less rapidly at increasing ranges. The intensity of these two types of echo may vary by as much as 80 dB when detected by an extracorporeal receiver. In the head the echoes from the brain are further attenuated in propagating across the skull by 20–40 dB. As a result, the low intensity scattered reflexions from the cellular discontinuities in the brain are so greatly attenuated that they cannot be detected above the noise level of the receiving system. The important consequence of this is that it is only possible to display the high amplitude specular reflexions from the surfaces of the brain and its ventricles by an ultrasonic reflexion technique with an extracranial transducer [3.21].

3.1.a. The M-echo

When a reflexion technique uses the same transducer as both generator and receiver, the only interfaces that can return high amplitude specular reflexions to the generator-receiver are those that lie in the transducer axis and are orientated so as to be normal to this axis. The convolutional surfaces of the brain or the walls of the lateral or third ventricles comprise interfaces separating the brain from CSF. Reflexions of high amplitude may arise from any of these interfaces which can be displayed by a pulse-echo technique so that their range can be

35

measured from their propagation time. In the cerebral midline there is a large number of such interfaces formed by the convolutions in the interhemispheric fissure and by the lateral walls of the third ventricle and the medial walls of the lateral ventricles. These interfaces are not totally planar but they all have parts of their surfaces which are co-planar with the median sagittal plane. Thus their echoes can be received by a generator-receiver, the axis of which is normal to the sagittal plane, *i.e.*, lies in the bitemporal axis. Moreover in the bitemporal axis all these interfaces in the cerebral median plane lie at approximately the same range so that, if they are displayed by an A-mode technique, the echoes from the different interfaces are superimposed and summate. For this reason the aggregate echoes from the cerebral median plane have a greater amplitude when displayed from the transtemporal axis than echoes from any other region of the brain. This is one of the properties of the M-echo by which it can be distinguished from the echoes from other cerebral interfaces [3.24, 3.25]

The interfaces, which in aggregate give rise to the M-echo, do not in practice all lie at the same position along the bitemporal axis. The interfaces mostly are in the hemispheres on either side of the interhemispheric fissure or the two walls of the third ventricle and thus lie in two groups each a millimetre or so to one or other side of the geometrical median plane. For this reason the aggregate of echoes comprising the M-echo is not only of high amplitude but also is characteristically twin peaked. It is this shape that has resulted in the aggregate echo being called the M-echo.

In cases of cerebral swelling the interhemispheric fissure tends to be obliterated and the interfaces on either side of it are pressed together. As a result the number of separate interfaces comprising the M-echo is reduced so that its amplitude declines. For the same reason the twin peaks of the M-echo tend to approximate and are no longer separately identifiable. Since it is only by its higher amplitude than other cerebral echoes and by its characteristic twin-peaked shape that the M-echo can be identified, this becomes more difficult in cases of cerebral swelling. When the cerebral swelling is accompanied by displacement and distortion of the midline interfaces so that many of them no longer lie normal to the beam, the identification of the M-echo is even more difficult. It is for this reason that most unsatisfactory midline examinations and errors are made in cases of cerebral swelling with or without displacement of the cerebral midline.

If an isolated brain is placed in a water tank and a search is made with a transducer at normal incidence to its sagittal plane, it is found that the M-echo is present throughout this plane but is of highest amplitude when the transducer axis transects the *anterior* region of the third ventricle [3.25]. This region lies at the centre of the incisura in the falx cerebri which restrains much of the cerebral hemisphere from being displaced laterally. Thus when deforming cerebral disease is present the anterior part of the third ventricle becomes displaced first and more than the other midline structures. It would be very helpful if midline echoencephalography could measure the position of the midline structures in this region. Unfortunately this is not possible and the high reflectivity of the skull is the reason.

There is a greater difference in the acoustic impedance between the skull and the soft tissues of the scalp and brain than for any other non-air-containing pair of tissues in the body. Thus, even at normal incidence, the skull reflects much of the energy that strikes it. The proportion of energy reflected increases with oblique incidence until, at the critical angle of 27° of incidence, all of the energy striking the skull is reflected and none can propagate across it. The consequence of this high reflectivity of the skull is that, if the maximal intensity of the generated sound is to propagate across the skull to insonate the brain, the generated energy must strike the skull at normal incidence, *i.e.*, the face of the transducer must be tangential to the skull. In exactly the same way, if the echoes reflected from the brain are to propagate across the skull at optimal intensity for extracranial detection, they too must strike the inner table of the skull at normal incidence. When these two requirements are combined with the fact that a generator-receiver can only detect specular echoes from interfaces which are normal to the beam, it can be appreciated that it is only possible to display, at optimal amplitude, echoes from interfaces lying in the median sagittal plane by placing the generator-receiver on that one region of the skull which lies parallel

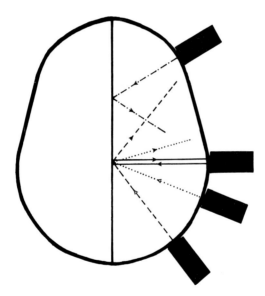

Fig. 3.1 Diagrammatic illustration that, if the transducer face must be tangential to the skull so that maximal amounts of energy may propagate both ways across the skull, specular reflexions from interfaces in the median sagittal plane only are returned to the generator-receiver when it is placed on the one region of the skull parallel to the median sagittal plane.

to this plane, as shown in Fig. 3.1. This is the widest part of the skull and, in most persons, it is just above the attachment of the ear to the scalp [3.19]. It can further be appreciated that, when the generator-receiver is correctly placed and aligned in this position to detect echoes from the median sagittal plane, it is also best placed and aligned to receive high amplitude echoes from the far side of the skull. This is illustrated in Fig. 3.2.

When the transducer is placed in this position and orientated with its axis

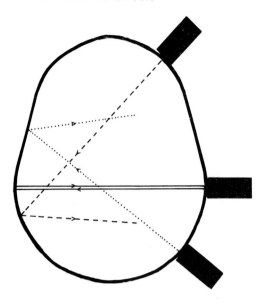

Fig. 3.2 Diagrammatic illustration that the same placement of the transducer necessary for echoes
from the median sagittal plane optimally to be displayed (Fig. 3.1) is also the placement
where echoes from the far side of the skull and scalp-air interface are optimally displayed.

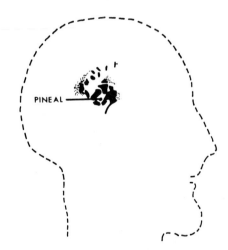

PINEAL

Fig. 3.3 Diagrammatic representation of the various interfaces in the median longitudinal fissure
and the third ventricular walls posteriorly, which lie close to the axis of the cone from which
echoes from interfaces in the median sagittal plane (Figs. 3.1 and 3.4) can be optimally
displayed. These are the interfaces that contribute, in varying degrees, to the M-echo
aggregate.

normal to the median sagittal plane, its axis transects this plane in the region of
the pineal gland [3.24]. It is for this reason that the interfaces that comprise the
M-echo which can be optimally displayed by an extracranial receiver arise from
the midline structures in the region of the pineal gland and *posterior* third
ventricle (see Fig. 3.3), and not from the preferable region of the *anterior* third

ventricle. At the same time the echoes from the far side of the head are also optimally displayed when the transducer is in its correct position and orientation for the display of the M-echo.

It can be appreciated that since this optimal placement and orientation of the transducer for the display of the M-echo is imposed upon the echoencephalographer by the laws of acoustics and the acoustical properties of the skull, the echoencephalographer has no control over them. If, in his frustrated desire to display the M-echo from other regions of the cerebral midline, he places the transducer on other regions of the skull and with other orientations, the result

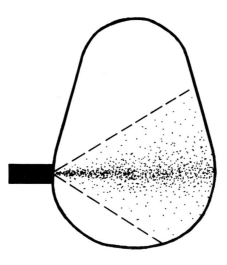

Fig. 3.4 The critical angle for total reflexion at a soft tissue-skull interface is 27°. The laws of refraction ensure that energy that has propagated through biplanar regions of skull must lie within this angle, *i.e.* within a cone with an apical angle of 54°. Within this cone the energy is distributed with varying intensity: the highest intensity is in the region of the axis (dense stippling) and the lowest intensity is near the edges of the cone (sparse stippling). This gradation in the distribution of the energy is not regular: scattering caused by the skull results in an irregular distribution.

   This same diagram can be used to represent the amplitude of the energy detected by an extracranial receiver from echoes of constant intensity from various regions of the brain. The amplitude is highest (dense stippling) when the echoes originate from the region of the axis of the cone and decreases from regions near the edge. No echoes can be detected by the extracranial receiver from interfaces lying outside the cone.

   Thus the same interfaces that are insonated by the highest intensities of energy from an extracranial generator are positioned so that they reflect echoes of optimal amplitude for detection by an extracranial receiver. This is the reason that the use of the same transducer as both generator and receiver is so advantageous.

must always be a degradation of the display. Since, as is described in the next Section, the display of the M-echo is none too easy, especially in cases of cerebral swelling, even with optimal placement and orientation of the transducer, such degradation is to be avoided.

3.1.b. The variability of the amplitude of the M-echo

The laws of refraction ensure that the energy that propagates through biplanar regions of the skull must be confined within a cone whose boundaries are determined by the critical angle for total reflexion [3.22]. Therefore it has an apical angle of 54° (2 × 27°). Within this cone the energy is distributed with varying intensities, as indicated in Fig. 3.4, with least intensity internal to the walls and highest intensity in the axis. Propagation through the skull, however, results in the energy not being distributed with its intensity varying regularly between these two extremes. The energy is very irregularly scattered in propagating through the skull so that its distribution within the cone is always very irregular [3.22] although showing a tendency to decline in amplitude in the more peripheral regions of the cone. Therefore it is apparent that a collection of interfaces such as give rise to the M-echo, as shown in Fig. 3.3, are insonated by quite variable intensities of energy so that their composite echo also varies markedly in amplitude.

The irregular scattering of the energy by the skull varies markedly in its distribution with any small movement of the beam relative to the skull [3.26]. The necessity to ensure that the transducer face is always tangential to the irregular contours of the skull, if maximal amplitudes of energy are to propagate both ways across the skull, can best be achieved when the transducer is held by hand and its face pressed flat onto the skull. It is difficult and undesirable to hold the transducer completely still for periods, so that the pattern of the irregularly scattered energy insonating the brain continually changes. As a result the amplitude of the M-echo and all other intracranial echoes is also continuously changing.

As a consequence, although the aggregate of echoes from the cerebral midline that comprise the M-echo often does give rise to an echo of greater amplitude than that of other intracerebral echoes and often this may be of characteristic twin-peaked shape, *this is not always the case throughout the echoencephalographic examination.* It is for this reason that it is undesirable that the transducer be held completely still during an echoencephalographic examination. If it is moved slightly throughout the examination the irregularities in the distribution of the isonating energy due to the skull become randomized. Under these circumstances although the M-echo may not be the echo of maximal amplitude at any one moment, over a period during which the distribution of the energy is randomized throughout the brain, it most often is the echo of maximal amplitude. Obviously, however, during this period of randomization its amplitude varies widely. It is this evanescence and variability in the display of the M-echo that is the cause of the greatest difficulty in midline echoencephalography.

3.1.c. Midline echoencephalographic techniques

There are two techniques whereby the midline echoencephalographic examination can be carried out: these are the conventional technique with a video display and the statistical technique whereby a large number of measurements is made automatically.

In the conventional technique the identification of the M-echo is made by the operator from the A-scan display. In many cases, especially in normal patients, this identification is relatively easy and requires little skill. In some patients, however, especially those with cerebral swelling, the identification of the M-echo is much more difficult. The problem that arises in such cases results from the evanescence of the A-mode display of the echoes from cerebral interfaces at all ranges along the time-base; because the operator is holding the transducer(s) and watching the video display that is, to some extent, under his control. With patience it is quite possible to manipulate the display so that an echo is seen which might be the M-echo at almost any distance along the time base. Every laboratory has examples of this fact though few are reported in the literature. Sandok *et al.* [3.13] reported an example where three normal echograms were obtained from a patient by an operator who did not realize that clinically a displaced cerebral midline was probable; when the examination was repeated by an operator aware of the clinical condition, the expected midline displacement was shown in three further echograms. From our laboratory we reported a case [3.22] in which the operator, aware that a temporal tumour had been diagnosed clinically, found a large displacement whereas the angiogram showed that the tumour was so diffusely invasive that it had not displaced the midline structures. We also reported [3.31] the results of re-reading 484 echoencephalograms in all of which the position of the cerebral midline had been confirmed by contrast radiography. When these echograms were re-read by a neurologist under strictly controlled conditions such that they could not be linked to either patient or diagnosis, he made an average of three false negative errors in each of four re-readings. Yet when he had read these echograms in their original clinical setting, he had not made a single false-negative error. Even though he had no contact with most of the patients examined, it is obvious that he had gained sufficient information, by indirect methods, to enable him to avoid making erroneous interpretations. Moreover when presented with the echograms on which he had made the errors on re-reading, he was unable to justify, from the echogram, the originally correct interpretation. Therefore, it is also obvious that, under certain circumstances, he had paid more attention to the indirectly acquired clinical information than to the echogram.

From these observations it is apparent that, if the greatest degree of accuracy is to be achieved by conventional midline echoencephalography, the examination must be carried out by an operator who can bias the echograms he records and his interpretation of them, by his own clinical knowledge of the patient's illness and whether or not the cerebral midline structures are likely to be displaced and, if so, to which side and by how much. It is for this reason that the greatest accuracy is achieved by the technique when it is carried out by a neurologist or neurosurgeon or under his close supervision. For the same reason Schiefer *et al.* [3.14], who have achieved the highest degree of accuracy with this technique, insist that 'the investigator must be informed on the entire clinical case through a knowledge of the history and the clinical findings and possess adequate knowledge on the pathological-anatomical relationships in intracranial disorders such as space-occupying and atrophic lesions. This can hardly be expected of paramedical personnel'.

If it is essential that the midline echoencephalographic examination, especially in difficult cases, must be carried out by a neurological specialist who has first made an examination of the patient and his records which is sufficient to form a presumptive diagnosis, some persons have questioned the economics of such an examination [3.20]. It would seem that the presumptive diagnosis contains more information than merely the finding of the position of the midline structures and this information is being acquired solely to improve the accuracy of the midline examination and then discarded. It would seem that the neurological specialist could better employ his hard acquired clinical skills.

This in no way should be interpreted as a criticism of the accuracy that has been achieved by certain echoencephalographers with the A-scan technique. The highest accuracy so far achieved has been in two large series of neurosurgical patients reported by Ford [3.2] and Schiefer et al. [3.14]. In both series the proportion of cases, with cerebral swelling with or without midline displacement, was higher than in most other reported series. Therefore such series contained more difficult examinations than other series, for example those reported by White [3.18], in which the percentage of cases with cerebral disease was much lower. Nevertheless, despite the greater difficulty of the cases they examined both Ford and, more particularly, Schiefer et al., achieved an amazing degree of accuracy; it was over 99 per cent in the series compiled by the latter. However Ford and Schiefer's colleague, Kazner, were employed as surgical registrar and Oberartz respectively at hospitals with very large neurosurgical populations; therefore they were directly responsible for the diagnosis and management of all the patients in their respective hospitals. As such they, of necessity, had to acquire detailed knowledge of the clinical condition of those patients whether or not they used this knowledge additionally to bias the echoencephalographic examination towards increased accuracy. It is only in the large neurosurgical clinics in Europe that the Oberartz or registrar spends many years in a position of immediate responsibility for large numbers of patients with cerebral diseases. In this way, not only does he have the time to develop and exercise the necessary echoencephalographic skills as an ancillary to his clinical skills, but he also has the opportunity to impart these skills to his assistants who stay an equally long time in such clinics. Thus his echoencephalographic examinations can be made by assistants almost as expert as he, when he is not present in the hospital or clinic. Such facilities are not present in North America where residents cannot acquire such a high degree of skill since no resident, with his intimate clinical knowledge of a large number of patients, ever stays in one position for five, ten or more years as does the Oberartz in Europe.

Moreover Ford and Kazner, who are both highly respected neurosurgeons, acquired their echoencephalographic skills by devoting much time to the technique when it was in its infancy. At that time its potentialities were unknown and were developed largely as a result of their efforts. It is to be wondered whether, even in Europe where the registrar and Oberartz system would favour such a development, young men would now be willing to devote the time necessary in order to emulate the skills of their predecessors with a technique the potential of which is now well understood.

It is on account of these reservations, concerning the willingness of another generation of echoencephalographers to follow in the footsteps of Ford and Kazner, that the automatic techniques have been developed [3.29]. The automatic techniques measure the range of the highest amplitude echo in the transtemporal axis many times. Since the highest amplitude echo is most often that of the M-echo, the median or the mode of the large number of measurements made indicates the position of the cerebral midline. Since there is no A-scan display, it is difficult for the operator to bias the results obtained. Thus no clinical skill is necessary to manipulate and bias the display in difficult cases and the examination can be carried out by a technician and does not depend for accuracy upon the close supervision of a neurological specialist.

3.1.d. The conventional technique with an A-scope

The echoencephalographer who uses the conventional technique must always remember that the accuracy that he achieves, especially in difficult cases where the need for accuracy is greatest, largely depends upon his clinical knowledge of the patient he is examining. This not only implies that the examination should be made by, or closely supervised by, a neurological specialist but also that it must be preceded by an examination of the patient's records and perhaps supplemented by interrogation and clinical examination of the patient. Before starting the

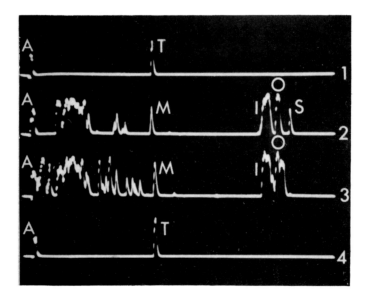

Fig. 3.5 A four level display of an undisplaced cerebral midline. The top and bottom traces show transmission pulses (T) across the head indicating the position of the geometrical midline. The two middle traces show that the two M-echoes are both equidistant from the transducers (AA) and at the same range as the transmission pulses. Therefore, the M-echoes are undisplaced from the geometrical midline.

These echograms illustrate the advantage of using transmission pulses to indicate the position of the geometrical midline. If the geometrical midline is calculated by halving the distance from the transducer (A) to the scalp-air interface (0) it is found to be displaced by half the depth to which the transducer face is indented below the surface of the scalp. Moreover it may not always be easy to distinguish the opposite scalp-air interface (0) from the reflexion from the inner table of the skull (T) nor from a reverberation echo between the opposite scalp-air interface and outer table of the skull (S).

examination, the echoencephalographer should have clearly in his mind the position where he expects to find the cerebral midline.

It is equally important that the display of the echoencephalograph should facilitate the operator's manipulation of the transducers best to demonstrate the position of the M-echo with respect to the median plane. For this purpose a multi-trace display is mandatory. The echoes from both sides of the head must be simultaneously displayed. At the same time the position of the geometrical midline of the head must be simultaneously displayed by one or two transmission pulses. Only with such a three or four trace display is the operator able to appreciate at a glance whether he is displaying simultaneously from both sides of the head echoes which resemble the M-echo in amplitude and shape and are at appropriate positions along the time-base. When the cerebral midline is undisplaced, the two M-echoes both appear at the same distance along the time base and also at the same distance along the time-base as the transmission pulse(s), as shown in Fig. 3.5. When the midline is displaced, the M-echoes must appear

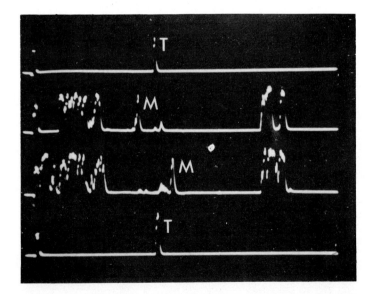

Fig. 3.6 A four level display similar to Fig. 3.5, but showing a displaced cerebral midline. The M-echoes (M) are displaced equidistant to either side of the geometrical midline indicated by the transmission pulses (T).

equidistant to either side of the transmission pulse (see Fig. 3.6). With such a display the operator's task is simplified in looking for and in displaying echoes at positions where his previous clinical examination tells him they are most likely to appear.

For the reasons already described, the examination is conducted by applying the transducers so that their faces are flat upon the scalp in the position where the head is widest, which is just above the ear. Their axes must be pointed at each other and, when they are symmetrically insonating those regions of the brain where the M-echo can be optimally displayed, this correct placement and orientation of the transducers is manifest on the display by the appearance of high amplitude echoes from the inner table of the opposite side of the skull and the overlying scalp-air interface at the same distance along the two time-bases and at approximately twice the distance of the transmission pulses, as shown in Figs. 3.5 and 3.6. Only when these criteria have been fulfilled is it permissible to start searching for the two M-echoes by manipulating the transducers until they are satisfactorily displayed. When they are so displayed it may be required that a permanent record of them be made by photography. Such a photograph is necessary when a displacement of the midline is present as its amount can be more easily measured at leisure from a photograph than directly from the display.

Table 3.1. Performance figures in A-scan echoencephalography.

Author	Year	Total number of cases	Unsatisfactory number	per cent	False +ve number	per cent	False −ve number	per cent
de Vlieger and Ridder	1959	34	0/34	0	?1/20	?5	2/14	14
Taylor et al.	1961	246	12/246	5	1/87	1	17/147	12
Lithaender and Marions	1961	252	8/252	3	1/83	1	16/161	10
Jeppson	1961	432	0/432	0	2/191	1	10/241	4
Jefferson	1962	229	3/229	1	7/67	10	13/159	8
Ford and Ambrose	1963	867	0/867	0	29/326	9	24/541	5
Russo and Arnold	1964	121	0/121	0	2/22	9	0/99	0
Lee and Morley	1964	77	0/77	0	3/77	4	3/44	7
Greebe	1964	671	6/250	2	6/?	?	11/?	?
Brinker et al.	1965	287	0/287	0	7/58	12	1/229	0·5
Lapayowker and Christen	1965	358	0/358	0	7/51	14	5/307	2
Raskind	1965	600	?	?	6/28	21	2/572	0·5
Kessler	1965	103	0/103	0	2/25	8	3/78	4
Barrows et al.	1965	159	0/159	0	1/43	2	8/116	7
McGinnis and Zylak	1965	795	88/795	11	1/20	5	1/364	0·25
Hagemann	1965	827	22/827	3	9/141	6	11/326	3
Hanson and Holmes	1966	200	7/200	3	5/16	31	1/23	4
Dugdale	1966	200	8/200	4	1/39	2	2/79	3
Blatt	1966	330	0/330	0	2/95	2	25/235	11
Gokalp et al.	1966	295	0/295	0	1/?	?	10/?	?
Fischer et al.	1967	1000	4/1000	0·5	4/248	2	8/748	1
Nichols et al.	1968	200	0/200	0	3/46	6	6/138	4
Brownbill and Dugdale	1968	269	10/269	4	6/45	12	7/214	3
Schiefer et al.	1968	1870	18/3140	0·5	15/844	2	3/?1008	0·33
White (original)	1969	484	57/484	12	10/31	32	0/396	0
White (revised)	1969	484	38/484	8	11/25	44	3/408	1

Notes.

Errors are confirmed cases only.

Percentages are approximated.

References are cited in the reference sections of [3.20, 3.28, 3.29, 3.32].

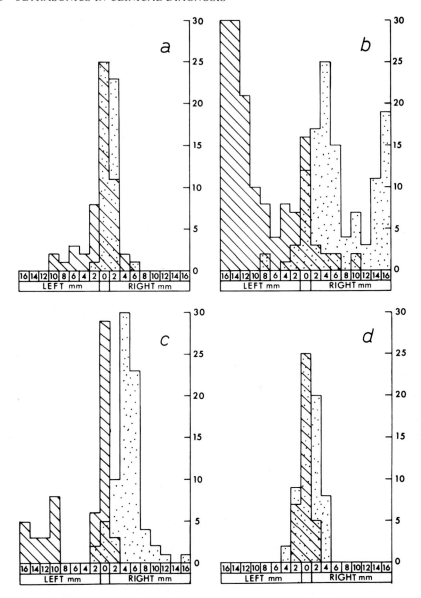

Fig. 3.7 Four histograms made on the same patient with the *Automatic Midline Computer*. The patient had suffered a moderately severe head injury and the histograms were made 1 h (*a*), 18 h (*b*), 25 h (*c*) and 72 h (*d*) afterwards. The patient's cerebral midline can be assumed not to have been displaced during this period.

(*a*) and (*d*) show that either the median or the mode of the histogram is easily identified and shows no shift is present.

This is not the case in (*b*) when cerebral swelling was maximal and, as a consequence, the high amplitude of the M-echo was reduced making it more difficult to identify by its amplitude from the echoes of other cerebral interfaces. It is for this reason all midline echoencephalographic techniques make more unsatisfactory examinations and more errors in cases of cerebral swelling with or without midline displacement.

Readings made with the transducer on the left temporal area are cross-hatched; those with the transducer on the right temporal area are stippled.

The accuracy achieved with the conventional technique varies quite widely from centre to centre, as indicated in Table 3.1. It is apparent that one reason for this is the variation in the amount of clinical bias that is used in different centres. Not all echoencephalographers are able or willing to supervise and, when necessary, bias the technique in order to achieve the accuracy of Schiefer *et al.* [3.14]. Another reason is the percentage of difficult cases with cerebral swelling in the series examined. It is much easier to achieve a high degree of accuracy when most of the patients examined are normal, and the technique is easiest.

3.1.e.   The automatic techniques

Two automatic devices are now commercially available. The Automatic Midline Computer* has been on the market for several years and its performance reasonably well evaluated [3.28]. Its mode of operation is to search for two high amplitude echoes from the far side of the head following the generation of the first pulse in a sequence. In this way it satisfies the requirement that the M-echo is best displayed when high amplitude echoes are also received from the far side of the head. If a satisfactory 'double distal' echo is received its propagation time is measured and halved. The corresponding range equals the range of of the geometrical midline of the head. A gate corresponding to a range of 16 mm of soft tissue is set to either side of this half propagation time and, following the generation of the next pulse, the propagation time of any single echo within this gate that exceeds a pre-set threshold amplitude is measured. The propagation time of this echo is compared with the half-propagation time of the double-distal echo and is displayed automatically as originating from an interface in the geometrical midline or so many millimetres to one or other side of the geometrical midline. The next measurement must be initiated by pressing a re-set button. A number of measurements are made and plotted on a histogram. Since the maximal amplitude echo is most often the M-echo, the median or mode of the histogram indicates the position of the cerebral midline. This is illustrated in Fig. 3.7.

The examination is carried out in the same way as with the video technique but, of course, does not need to be preceded by a clinical examination of the patient. It can be performed by a technician since it is almost impossible to bias or influence the measurements it makes. It is apparent that before a measurement can be made, the logic of the device must be satisfied that the transducer is correctly placed and aligned so that high amplitude far side echoes are received. While this is an excellent safeguard against misuse, it is responsible for some drawbacks to the technique. In the presence of cerebral swelling, as already described, all techniques have greater difficulty in identifying the M-echo since its amplitude is reduced. This applies equally to the automatic techniques. In such cases the Midline Computer may find it difficult to set the mid-gate and measurements may be made only very slowly or, sometimes, not at all. Under these circumstances the operator may start moving the transducer to a position where measurements are more readily made. If the transducer should be moved upwards and backwards from its correct position echoes may be obtained from

*Diagnostic Electronics Corporation, Box 580, Lexington, MA 02173, USA.

the falx cerebri. Since the falx cerebri is relatively rigid and is little displaced in deforming cerebral disease, a false negative error may be made [3.28]. When difficulty is encountered in setting the mid-gate and the measurements are made slowly or with much scatter, it is posible to operate the Midline Computer in a two-transducer mode. In this way the mid-gate is set by means of a transmission pulse. Measurements are made faster and the histograms show less scatter.

Table 3.2. Performance figures in automated echoencephalography.

Author	Instrument	Year	Total no. of cases	Unsatisfactory		False +ve		False −ve	
				number	per cent	number	per cent	number	per cent
Hopman et al.	AMC	1973	530	34/530	6	6/114	5	3/382	1
Brisman et al.	AMC	1974	135	16/135	12	1/25	4	2/15	13
Klinger et al.	AMC	1974	1889	344/1886	18	33/434	8	11/1100	1
White and Hanna	AMC	1975	6667	183/6667	2·7	84−102/505	17−20*	13−18/5979	0·2−0·3
Hudson and Müller	DE	1974	150	4/150	3	1/18	5	0/59	0

Notes
  *12 per cent of the *patients* examined and found to have shifts were false positive errors.
  AMC: Automatic Midline Computer; DE: Digiecho.
  Percentages are approximated.
  References are cited in the reference sections of [3.28, 3.32].

The Midline Computer compares favourably in accuracy with the A-scan technique (see Table 3.2), except in those few centres where the A-scan examination is carried out under the close supervision of the neurological specialist using his clinical skills to achieve the highest accuracy.

In one series of cases examined with the Midline Computer (Klinger et al. [3.7]) a very high percentage of unsatisfactory examinations was made, as recorded in Table 3.2. This series was compiled by the very same German centres which have achieved such a high degree of accuracy with the A-scan technique. Since Klinger et al. have concluded that this high percentage of unsatisfactory examinations makes the automatic technique unsuitable for use in the case of neurosurgical emergencies, which are the very cases in which White and Hannah [3.28] have found it to be most helpful, it may be worthwhile to examine more closely the causes of the 18 per cent of unsatisfactory examinations in Klinger et al.'s series in contrast to the 2·7 per cent in the series reported by White and Hannah. Firstly, in each of the three hospitals used in Klinger et al.'s series the results obtained by the Midline Computer were compared, for accuracy, with a subsequent examination with the A-scan technique. Where the two results differed the A-scan result was assumed to be correct, and the Midline Computer, to be in error. Therefore there cannot have been much incentive to complete the examination with the Midline Computer satisfactorily. In White and Hannah's series, however, the only echoencephalographic examination made was that with the Midline Computer, so there was very great pressure upon the operator concerned to complete the examination satisfactorily more especially as the neurosurgeons, have learnt to trust the accuracy of the result, were eager to hear whether a midline shift was present or not, as their subsequent management of the patient depended importantly upon this factor. Secondly, in one of the hospitals used in Klinger *et al.*'s series, students were used with no training or knowledge of echoencephalography. While the automatic techniques can be successfully used by persons without the high degree of clinical and echoencephalographic skill necessary for the A-scan technique, they cannot be used successfully by persons with no training at all. The effect of such unskilled operators is shown by Klinger *et al.*'s finding that 29 per cent of the first 150 cases examined by such an operator were unsatisfactory or erroneous while only 8 per cent were unsatisfactory or erroneous in the second 150 cases examined by the same operator. Thirdly, at the Munich hospital used in Klinger *et al.*'s series, an arbitrary time limit was imposed upon the automatic technique. If it appeared that the examination would not be completed in 10 minutes or less, then it was terminated and called unsatisfactory. The reason for this time limit is that the large neurosurgical clinic at Munich is equipped to deal so promptly with neurosurgical emergencies that, when necessary, a craniotomy or diagnostic angiogram can be commenced within 10 minutes of the patient's admission. Therefore 10 minutes is all the time available for echoencephalography at Munich. The Kingston hospital on the other hand, used for White and Hannah's series, is a general hospital in which the personnel and space necessary for cerebral angiograms and craniotomies are not constantly available. Such procedures cannot be carried out in less than an hour following admission and therefore this longer time is available for echoencephalography. Since the measurements made by the Midline Computer are often much slower in cases of neurosurgical emergencies with cerebral swelling, many such cases require 30 or 40 minutes for the examination to be completed. Certainly the automatic techniques can never be used satisfactorily where a short and rigid time limit needs to be imposed.

The other automatic device is the Digiecho*. Although prototypes have been in use since 1973 their operation needed frequent small changes so that a standardized model was not developed until 1975. Moreover, prior to the granting of patent rights in 1975 neither the designer nor the manufacturer were willing to disclose the mode of operation of the device and had prevented the user from finding these out for himself by obliterating the identification marks on the components used. For these reasons it will be some years before the advantages and disadvantages of this automatic device can be as clearly understood as is the case with the Midline Computer.

The Digiecho is a simpler device than the Midline Computer and, because it was designed to be carried in the pocket, less robust. It was made so compact because the designer envisioned that the demand for midline echoencephalography was greatest at the bedside upon patients during the course of a neurological examination. In fact, the greatest demand for midline echoencephalography (see Section 3.1.f) appears to be in the emergency department where the advantages of a compact device are not great.

*Radionics Ltd., Montreal, Canada.

The Digiecho also differs from the Midline Computer in the fact that the geometrical centre of the head, with which the range of the maximal amplitude echo is compared, is not calculated afresh each time from the pulse preceding that from which the range of the echo is measured. The geometrical midline of the head is measured either by a pair of calipers or a one-way transmission pulse at the start of the examination and before the ranges of any echoes are measured. Following this measurement the gate is centred upon it manually by the operator. This is a simpler procedure than the automatic measurement of the range of the double distal echo by the Midline Computer and therefore simplifies the examination of those cases where the double distal echo is hard to elicit. It has the disadvantage, however, that it compares the range of the M-echo made with various placements of the transducer in the region of the pinna with a transmission range made from a single placement. Not only is the skull surface slightly irregular in the region above the ear, so that the range between two transducers varies slightly, but also the thickness of the bone in this region varies quite markedly so that variations in the transmission range measured occur, due to the energy propagating through varying thicknesses of the skull at about twice the velocity in soft tissue [3.27]. The magnitude of these two errors can be readily determined by making a series of measurements of transmission range between two transducers as they are slightly moved around the above-pinna placement. It is found that the transmission ranges measured vary through a range of 3—4 mm. For this reason it seems wisest that about a dozen measurements, instead of only one, of the transmission range should be made initially. Not only does this simplify the comparison of the range of echo-range measurements with the range of transmission-range measurements, but it constantly reminds the user of the ranging errors present in all midline echoencephalographic techniques [3.27].

After the gate is centred upon the median or mode of the transmission ranges measured, the device is switched to make measurements of the intracranial echoes. It generates a series of 60 or so pulses at a repetition rate of 60 s^{-1} in a period of 1·0 s. Throughout this period the amplification of the receiver is progressively increased at a rate approximating 1 dB between successive pulses, until an echo is received and amplified to a level in excess of a pre-set threshold. The range of this echo is then automatically displayed for about a second, during which the device is inactivated before the whole sequence restarts automatically. In addition to the slow increase in receiver gain between successive pulses, the amplification also increases a further 3 dB following the generation of each pulse in order to provide a type of time-gain compensation for the more greatly attenuated echoes from distant reflectors. The measurements made are plotted manually on a histogram but, unlike the Midline Computer, are not displayed as a range from the theoretical midline, but as a range from the transducer. Therefore the operator must determine whether these measurements indicate displacement of the midline structures or not. If the distribution curves are equidistant from the transducer when it is on either side of the head, the inference is that no shift is present. The transmission range provides a check upon these measurements and, when no shift is present, should be at the same range as the maximal amplitude echoes from the left and right side. When midline displacement is present the transmission range should be intermediate between those of

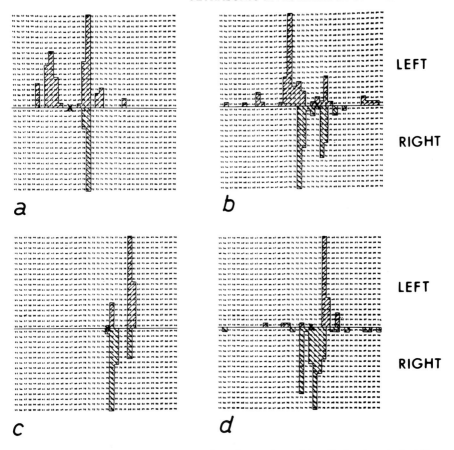

LEFT

RIGHT

LEFT

RIGHT

a   b

c   d

Fig. 3.8 Four histograms made by the *Digiecho* on four patients with undisplaced cerebral midlines and which show incongruity between the ranges of the transmission pulses (X) and of the echoes of maximal amplitude. The upper histograms are made with the transducer on the left side of the head and the lower when it is on the right.

In (a) the interpreter is not certain whether there is a 4 mm shift to the left or whether no shift is present but a ranging error has increased the range of the maximal amplitude echoes from both sides of the head by 4 mm over that of the transmission range. Their uncertainty is made the greater by knowledge of the operator's ability to increase the number of measurements made for an echo at one given range by holding the transducer still. The range of the echoes measured most often exceeds those of the transmission range (a, c, d).

Such uncertainties can be reduced when a number of transmission range measurements are made and their median calculated rather than a single measurement. For instance, in (a) if the median measurement for the transmission range was found to be 71 mm instead of 67 mm as indicated, the histogram could be read with some confidence as showing no displacement of the midline.

Unfortunately the measurement of several transmission ranges does not eliminate all such uncertainties and, in the four histograms of this illustration, the indicated transmission range (X) was the median from 12 transmission range measurements.

the echoes from each side. Unfortunately, quite often there is a discrepancy between the ranges of the echoes displayed and that of the transmission pulse (see Fig. 3.8). It would seem that, in such cases, the Digiecho is making a ranging error. All midline echoencephalographic techniques, both with a video display and the automatic techniques, are subject to such ranging errors [3.22, 3.27].

Some of these are due to the acoustic properties of the head and some to the signal processing of the device used. The Digiecho makes a constant correction, in the ranges it displays, based upon an estimate of the normal thickness of the adult skull. Since the discrepancy usually (but not always) results in echo ranges of greater magnitude than the transmission range, it would appear that the most likely cause of this defect is not the result of variations in skull thickness from the normal, but rather the registration of the range of off-axis echoes from the midline due to refraction of the beam by the inner table of the skull [3.22, 3.27].

Another important difference between the operation of the two automatic devices arises as a result of the simplicity of the mode of operation of the Digiecho. Since there is no far-side logic to satisfy, and each measurement is initiated automatically without the need manually to press a re-set button, it is very easy for the operator, by holding the transducer stationary on the head, to initiate a whole series of measurements of any one echo at a single range. Therefore, the accuracy of the Digiecho depends heavily upon the operator continually moving the transducer throughout the whole series of measurements made, in order to randomize irregularities in the intensity of the energy insonating all the cerebral interfaces so that the echoes from the cerebral midline are most often those of highest amplitude and measured. It is not so easy to ensure that the operator always follows these instructions since, if the movements of the transducer are too vigorous, the measurements are so widely scattered that it takes much longer to compile a valid distribution curve of the echo of maximal amplitude and, often, the histogram will contain so many scattered measurements that it cannot be satisfactorily interpreted.

Another important factor that must be borne in mind when using either of the automatic devices is the level at which the threshold is set for measuring the echo of maximal amplitude. There is an inverse relationship between the height of this threshold and the speed with which measurements are made; the lower the threshold the more frequently does the amplitude of a received echo exceed it. There is a direct relationship between the threshold level and the accuracy of the measurements; the higher the threshold the more likely it is that it is the composite echo from the midline structures that exceed it. Thus if an automatic device makes its measurements fast but compiles histograms with much scatter due to measuring the ranges of non-midline echoes, it should be suspected that the threshold is set too low. If its measurements are made inacceptably slowly, albeit with increased accuracy, the threshold may be too high.

Conventional A-scan techniques and both the automatic techniques make errors. These are most often made on patients with cerebral swelling as would be expected. Interestingly, when one technique makes such an error the other two usually make the same type of error as well. Therefore there would appear to be little significant difference in the accuracy of these various techniques. It is in the unsatisfactory examinations that the greatest differences arise. They too occur most frequently in cases of cerebral swelling. Not infrequently is an examination unsatisfactory with one technique and clearly interpretable with the other; this difference also applies to the two automatic techniques; one may provide a histogram that is readily interpretable while the other may not. It has been possible to understand the causes of most of the unsatisfactory examinations made with the Midline Computer [3.28]; now that the mode of operation of the Digiecho has been disclosed, it may become possible to understand the causes of the unsatisfactory examinations made by it as well.

3.1.f.   Indications for midline echoencephalography

Until the recent development of automatic techniques with acceptable accuracy, midline echoencephalography was, of necessity, confined to neurological and neurosurgical centres because it was in these centres that the echoencephalographer, who had acquired the necessary expertise to bias the technique towards acceptable accuracy, worked. The development of automatic techniques has freed midline echoencephalography from this restriction. The technique can now be carried out in any centre. Therefore it is of some interest to determine in which clinical conditions the technique appears to be of greatest value. It seems that, even when the technique can now be used satisfactorily in any of a wide number of clinical settings, it proves still to be of most value and in greatest demand in the emergency department [3.28]—the same setting in which the clinical echoencephalographer developed the A-scan technique to such a high degree of accuracy.

Head injuries comprise by far the largest group of patients in which midline echoencephalography is of value to the clinician. Following a head injury, it may be very difficult to tell by clinical examination if intracranial bleeding is present with the necessity of early operation. Other conditions, such as unexplained coma or the recent onset of a stroke, less commonly require midline echoencephalography. Interestingly enough, midline echoencephalography appears to play only a small part in the investigation of the non-emergent, neurological problem. It was to enable the bedside examination of such patients that the Digiecho was designed in such a compact form. It appears, however, that the clinical or other technological examinations available for the diagnosis of such cases provide more valuable clinical information than a knowledge of the presence or absence of a midline shift. While such examinations are often made as part of the battery of tests to which all neurological patients are subject, rarely does the echoencephalographer find that the results of his examination are of much importance to the clinician. The situation is quite different in the emergency department where both clinical and other information is often lacking and hard to obtain in the patient presenting as a neurosurgical emergency. It is this paucity of information that makes midline echoencephalography so much more valuable in these cases and is the reason that the neurosurgeon often impatiently awaits to hear whether or not there is a midline shift in order to determine which form his management of the patient will take.

The need for midline echoencephalography in emergencies necessitates that the service should be available on a 24 h basis. This puts an intolerable strain upon the necessary neurological supervision in all but the biggest centres, if a conventional A-scan technique is used.

3.2 OTHER ECHOENCEPHALOGRAPHIC TECHNIQUES

3.2.a.   Ventriculography

The desire to display echoes from structures other than those of the cerebral midline, such as the walls of the third and lateral ventricles in order to measure ventricular size, arose naturally as a consequence of midline echoencephalography with an A-scan display. Therefore it is not surprising to find that those same echoencephalographers who developed midline echoencephalography to such a high degree of accuracy with the A-scan display, are the same as those who have developed echoventriculography. Schiefer *et al.* [3.14] and Ford [3.3] are the outstanding examples.

The difficulty with echoventriculography arises from the fact that the ventricular walls are often curved in complex shapes so that the area which is normal to the transducer axis is often small and therefore returns, by specular reflexion, an echo of relatively low amplitude. The exception is the third ventricle, the walls of which comprise large planar interfaces and which, in their posterior extent, contribute importantly to the M-echo complex. It is thus possible, by displaying these twin peaks, to measure the width of the third ventricle. It must be remembered, however, that, because of the high reflectivity of soft tissue-skull interfaces, even these high amplitude echoes from the third ventricular walls cannot be optimally displayed by an extracranial generator-receiver save in their posterior extent where they lie parallel to the overlying skull (see Section 3.1.a).

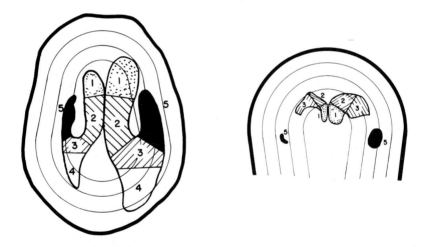

Fig. 3.9 Diagrammatic horizontal (left) and coronal (right) sections through the lateral ventricles. The lateral ventricles are of normal size on the left of each figure and dilated on the right. The lines drawn within the skull represent the loci of the ideal orientation for ventricular interfaces which can reflect an echo that can be optimally displayed by a generator-receiver the face of which is tangential to the overlying skull.

The walls of parts 1, 2 and 5 of the ventricular system are aligned such that their echoes can best be displayed by an extracranial transducer and larger areas of these walls are optimally aligned when the ventricles are dilated (see Section 3.2.*a*.).

This restriction also applies to the echoes from the walls of the lateral ventricles. Fig. 3.9 shows that there are only certain regions in which the walls of the lateral ventricles lie parallel to the overlying skull, and therefore can give rise to specular echoes which are optimally displayed extracranially. For this reason most attempts to display echoes from the lateral ventricles are confined to the frontal horns at the junction of parts 1 and 2; from the body of the ventricle (part 2) and the temporal horn (part 5). The temporal horn lies inferiorly and close to the surface so that it can only be displayed from the opposite side of the head to avoid undue inclination of the transducer on the surface of the scalp and the reverberation echoes between the transducer and skull which obscure the display of superficial echoes from the brain.

Fig. 3.9 also shows that, when the lateral ventricles dilate, their walls more closely approximate to a parallel orientation to the overlying skull and therefore echoes from them are more readily displayed. Of more importance, however, is the consequent enlargement of the area of the ventricular wall that lies normal to the transducer axis so that the specular reflexions from this region are increased in amplitude. It is much easier to display echoes from the walls of dilated lateral ventricles as a consequence. The display of these echoes is further enhanced in cases of ventricular dilatation since the ventricular fluid is anechoic so that, in an A-mode display, echoes from the walls of the ventricles arise from an anechoic baseline to one side.

Finally the same scattering of the energy that propagates across it by the skull and which is responsible for the variability in the amplitude of the M-echo as a result of small movements of the transducer with respect to the skull, also is responsible for variations in the amplitude of the echoes from the ventricular walls making them difficult to identify. The skulls of babies scatter the energy to a much smaller degree.

As a result of all these factors, echoventriculography in varying circumstances comprises a vast spectrum of difficulty. At the one extreme, the display and measurement of lateral ventricular width in hydrocephalic babies is so easy that it can readily be learned, and Sjögren [3.15, 3.16] is justified in calling it an easy and accurate technique. At the other extreme, the measurement of the size of undilated lateral ventricles in adults is so difficult and inaccurate [3.23] that it can probably never be a useful examination. It is for this reason that Kazner and Hopman [3.6], who are probably more expert in this field than anyone else, do not attempt to measure lateral ventricular size in adults unless they have previously demonstrated, by means of the easier third ventricular width measurement, that the third ventricle is enlarged so that the lateral ventricles are also likely to be enlarged. In between these extremes echoventriculography varies in difficulty and accuracy; the technique is more difficult in children than in babies, and in adults than in children; undilated ventricles always are more difficult to display than dilated ventricles and the lateral ventricles than the posterior portion of the third ventricle. The echoencephalographer who devotes much time and skill to the procedure becomes better at it than the casual echoencephalographer, and able to examine successfully more difficult cases. It is to be wondered, however, as was the case with midline echoencephalography, whether future echoencephalographers will have the facilities and be willing to devote the time and skill necessary to emulate the expertise acquired by Kazner and Ford.

Even if echoventriculography in adults should prove too difficult and demanding for the average echoencephalographer, it seems unfortunate that present disillusionment with the technique has also led to its neglect in the examination of babies. The presence or absence of hydrocephalus is important clinical information in the examination of babies and so is the periodic measurement of ventricular width during the treatment of hydrocephalus. In babies the examination is so much easier that most persons should be able to acquire the necessary skills.

3.2.b.   Transdural echoencephalography

All the tribulations of the echoencephalographer arise from the acoustic properties of the skull. When the skull is removed at operation he really comes into his own [3.9]. It is then readily possible to display the ventricular walls and, if necessary, to advise the neurosurgeon in which direction and to what depth his

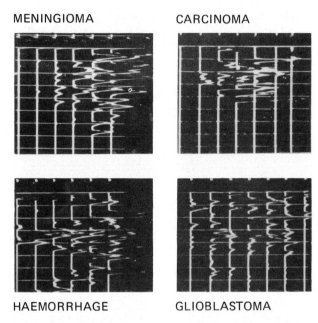

Fig. 3.10 A single photograph from each of four separate cases examined by transdural echoencephalography. Each photograph contains six or seven A-mode scans from different positions equidistant along a horizontal line projected on the dura mater exposed at operation.

It may be noted that the meningioma and secondary carcinoma, which are circumscribed tumours with sharp boundaries, show these features with well defined boundaries in their echograms from which echoes of regularly high amplitude are recorded. The fact that the meningioma extends to the surface can be appreciated, as can the completely intracerebral location of the metastasis.

The diffusely invasive glioblastoma, on the other hand, shows no well defined boundaries and, at its edges, the echoes tend to be of low and irregular amplitude.

The moderately well defined margins of the intracerebral haemorrhage can be appreciated and also, within its boundaries is an anechoic area consisting of liquid or clotted blood. Intracerebral cysts show similar anechoic regions. (*Courtesy*: H.R. Müller.)

brain needle must be passed in order to perform a ventricular puncture. It is equally easy to display intracerebral lesions, to estimate their size and position, and even to make an educated guess at their pathology. This is illustrated in Fig. 3.10. Too few neurosurgeons are aware of the help that echoencephalography can give them in helping them to find hard-to-localize lesions and in showing them the best routes and sites from which biopsy specimens can be obtained. At the same time as helping the neurosurgeon, the echoencephalographer will receive a boost to his own morale and be able to assure himself that it is true that valuable information can indeed be obtained from the brain by an ultrasonic reflexion technique.

3.2.c. Cerebral tomography

All the techniques described so far image only in the range dimension. The acoustical properties of the skull have, to date, defeated all attempts to make clinically useful two-dimensional ultrasonic images of the brain. The scattering of the energy by the skull results in more severe degradation of resolution in the lateral dimensions than in the range dimension. Cerebral tomograms succeed usually in displaying, with poor resolution, only echoes from part of the cerebral midline and part of the lateral ventricles. In babies these structures are more fully displayed and it is possible to obtain clinical information when structure is fairly grossly disturbed [3.8]. Cerebral tumours are not common in babies, however, although hydrocephalus is. Therefore, tomography is most useful in the diagnosis of hydrocephalus in babies [3.8].

Electronically scanned transducer arrays enable a scan to be completed in a fraction of a second. By making repeated scans a series of tomograms can be displayed in real time [3.17]. Such real time tomograms show no improvement in resolution* but they do have the advantage that they sometimes display echoes which can be seen to move synchronously with the cardiac pulse. Such echoes originate from the larger cerebral arteries and their display may indicate that the vessel is not thrombosed [3.4].

3.3 ECHOENCEPHALOGRAPHIC RANGING

Attempts have been made for many years to obtain clinical information from the fluctuations in the amplitude of intracranial echoes that occur synchronously with the cardiac pulse, respiration and other physiological variables. Such pulsatile echoencephalographic studies have not proved especially rewarding and have been shown to be prone to artifactual changes when a fixed gate is used [3.32], and not easily interpretable even when adequately recorded [3.1]. The one exception to this statement is the demonstration by Richardson *et al.* [3.12] that it is possible to record the plateau waves of raised intracranial pressure by this technique.

Since the variations in amplitude recorded in pulsatile echoencephalography result from movement of the interfaces of the brain, it seems more appropriate to record this movement directly. In this way many of the difficulties and restrictions of the amplitude recordings are avoided. Moreover additional information is acquired since the direction of movement is meaningful, while the direction of amplitude change is not.

In this way, it has been possible to show that, contrary to customary belief, the

---

*The use of a stationary transducer array alleviates some of the degradation due to probe movement which is inevitable with single-element transducers—editor.

ventricular system is compressed during the passage of the arterial pulse through the brain [3.30]. It is equally possible to record, by this non-invasive technique, the various pressure waves that occur in patients with raised intracranial pressure. This is illustrated in Fig. 3.11.

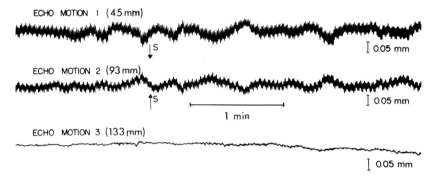

Fig. 3.11 Recording by echoencephalographic ranging of intracranial pressure waves in a patient with a cerebellar tumour. The top tracing records the variations in range of an interface at a depth of 45 mm in the ipsilateral hemisphere, the middle trace of an interface in the contralateral hemisphere. The bottom trace records the range of the opposite inner table of the skull at a distance of 133 mm and is included to ensure there is no movement of the transducer with respect to the skull that might cause artifact.

Upward deflexions of the pens represent increase in range, and *vice versa*. The arrows indicate the direction of motion that accompanies the propagation of the arterial pulse through the brain and represent the direction of motion of the interfaces that accompanies an increase in intracerebral volume and pressure. As is always the case, increased intracerebral volume causes centripetal motion of the two hemispheres.

The intracerebral pressure waves with a frequency of 2–3 min^{-1} are clearly seen superimposed upon the range changes due to the arterial pulse and to respiration at 23 min^{-1}.

3.4 DOPPLER TECHNIQUES

3.4.a.   Directional Doppler recording from the ophthalmic artery

Occlusion of the internal carotid artery is an important factor in the development of cerebrovascular disease. When it occurs, quite frequently it produces no symptoms. By the time symptoms develop the occlusion may have been present for many years and hence much less amenable to surgical correction.

The only artery that originates from the internal carotid artery before its termination at the base of the brain is the ophthalmic artery which supplies the eye and other tissues in the orbit before its terminal branches anastomose with branches of the external carotid artery over the forehead, and superficially and deep in the cheek. When the internal carotid artery is occluded, flow in the ophthalmic artery is reversed and the tissues in the orbit are supplied with blood by the external carotid artery. With a directional Doppler flowmeter it is easy to record the direction of flow in the ophthalmic artery and whether it be in the normal anterograde direction. When the flow is found to be reversed in this way (see Fig. 3.12) there is a very strong probability that the internal carotid artery on that side is either totally occluded, or has a significant stenosis of over 70 per cent of its lumen [3.10].

This is such a simple technique, with a fairly high degree of reliability, that neurologists should make more use of it.

3.4.b. Velocity tomography of the carotid bifurcation

If a directional beam is used it is possible to scan across the carotid bifurcation and to display congruously in the two lateral dimensions regions where the velocity of blood in vessels exceeds a pre-set threshold [3.11]. This technique can be used to display the velocity of blood flowing in the region of the carotid bifurcation where most occlusive disease occurs. Occlusion of one vessel is shown by its absence from the velocity tomogram. By raising the velocity threshold for display it is also possible to demonstrate the presence of a stenosis or partial occlusion by the high velocity jet that is associated with it. This is illustrated in Fig. 3.13.

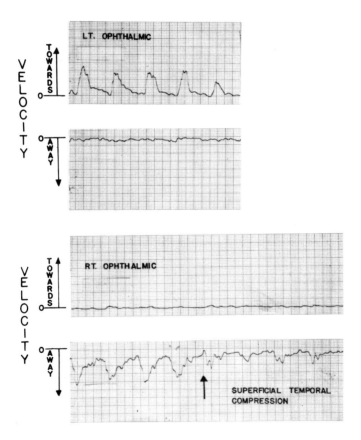

Fig. 3.12 Reversal of blood flow in the right ophthalmic artery recorded by a directional Doppler system in a case of occlusion of the right internal carotid artery. Normally the flow is towards the probe at the front of the orbit. The reversed flow comes from branches of the external carotid artery as shown by its reduction when the ipsilateral superficial temporal artery is compressed.

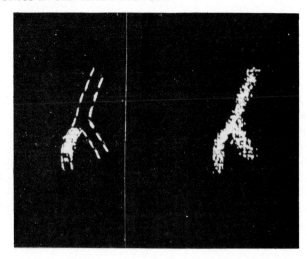

Fig. 3.13 Velocity tomogram of the carotid bifurcation in a patient with stenosis of the internal carotid artery. The tomogram on the left shows that flow is occurring in the common carotid artery and both its internal and external carotid branches.

    In the tomogram on the right, the velocity threshold for display has been raised and shows the high velocity jet at the origin of the internal carotid artery caused by a stenosis. The contours of the arterial bifurcation displayed with the lower threshold, have been outlined on this restricted display to help in spatial orientation.

REFERENCES

3.1. CLARK, J.M., WHITE, D.N., CURRY, G.R., STEVENSON, R.J., CAMPBELL, J.K. and JENKINS, C.O. (1971). The measurement of intracranial echo pulsations. *Med. biol. Engng.*, **9**, 263–87.

3.2. FORD, R.M. and AMBROSE, J. (1963). Echoencephalography: the measurement of the position of midline structures in the skull with high frequency ultrasound. *Brain*, **86**, 189–96.

3.3 FORD, R.M. and McRAE, D.L. (1966). Echoencephalography—a standardized technique for the measurement of the width of the third and lateral ventricles. In *Diagnostic Ultrasound*, Ed. C.C. Grossman, J.H. Holmes, C. Joyner and E.W. Purnell, pp. 117–29. New York: Plenum Press.

3.4 FREUND, H.J. (1974). Electronic sector scanning in cerebral diagnostics. 3. Visualization of intracranial structures and brain arteries. In *Ultrasonics in Medicine*, ed. M. de Vlieger, D. N. White and V. R. McCready, pp. 314–7. Amsterdam: Excerpta Medica.

3.5. JENKINS, C.O., CAMPBELL, J.K. and WHITE, D.N. (1971). Modulation resembling Traube-Hering waves recorded in the human brain. *Europ. Neurol.*, **5**, 1–6.

3.6. KAZNER, E. and HOPMAN, H. (1973). Possibilities and reliability of echoventriculography. *Ultrasound Med. Biol.*, **1**, 17–32.

3.7. KLINGER, M., KAZNER, E., GRUMME, TH., AMTENBRINK, V., GRAEF, G., HART-MANN, K.H., HOPMAN, H., MEESE, W. and VOGEL, B. (1975). Experience with automatic midline echoencephalography—a cooperative study of three neurosurgical clinics. *J. Neurol. Neurosurg. Psychiat.*, **38**, 272–8.

3.8. KOSSOFF, G., GARRETT, W.J. and RADAVANOVICH, G. (1974). Ultrasonic atlas of normal brain of infant. *Ultrasound Med. Biol.*, **1**, 259–66.

3.9. MÜLLER, H.R. (1971). *Die transdurale Echoenzephalographie.* Bern: Verlag Hans Huber.

3.10. MÜLLER, H.R. (1971). The diagnosis of internal carotid artery occlusion by directional Doppler sonography of the ophthalmic artery. *Neurology*, **22**, 816–23.

3.11. REID, J. M. and SPENCER, M.P. (1972). Ultrasound Doppler technique for imaging blood vessels. *Science, N.Y.*, **176**, 1235–6.

3.12. RICHARDSON, A., EVERSDEN, I.D. and STERNBERGH, W.C.A. (1972). Detecting intracranial pressure waves with ultrasound. *Lancet*, **i**, 355–7.

3.13. SANDOK, B.A., HENSON, T.E. and SKAGGS, H. (1970). Analysis of echoencephalograms: an evaluation of interpreter consistency. *Neurology*, **20**, 933–8.
3.14. SCHIEFER, W., KAZNER, E. and KUNZE, ST. (1968). *Clinical Echoencephalography*. New York: Springer-Verlag.
3.15. SJÖGREN, I. (1967). Echoencephalography in pediatric practice with special regard to measurement of the ventricular size. *Acta paed. scand.*, suppl. **178**, 1–67.
3.16. SJÖGREN, I. (1968). Echoencephalography in infants and children. *Acta radiol.*, suppl. **278**, 1–83.
3.17. SOMER, J.C. (1974). Electronic sector scanning in cerebral diagnostics. 1. Principle and technical development. In *Ultrasonics in Medicine*, Ed. M. de Vlieger, D.N. White and V.R. McCready, pp. 304–8. Amsterdam: Excerpta Medica.
3.18. WHITE, D.N. (1968). Amplitude averaged echoencephalography. In *Diagnostica Ultrasonica in Ophthalmologica*, pp. 93–100. Purkinje: University of Purkinje Press.
3.19. WHITE, D.N. (1970). The six 'laws' of echoencephalography. *Neurology*, **20**, 435–44.
3.20. WHITE, D.N. (1971). A-scan echo-encephalography at the crossroads: art or science? *Med. biol. Engng.*, **9**, 289–96.
3.21. WHITE, D.N. (1973). The sources of echoes displayed extracranially in echoencephalography. *Ultrasonics*, **11**, 263–7.
3.22. WHITE, D.N. (1976). *Ultrasonic Encephalography II*. Oxford: Pergamon Press.
3.23. WHITE, D.N. and BAHULEYAN, K. (1969). Restrictions of the A-scan echoencephalographic technique estimating lateral ventricular size. *Med. biol. Engng.*, **7**, 607–18.
3.24. WHITE, D.N., CLARK, J.M. and CAMPBELL, J.K. (1969). Inferential observations on the origin of the M-echo. *Med. biol. Engng.*, **7**, 481–91.
3.25. WHITE, D.N., CLARK, J.M., CAMPBELL, J.K., CHESEBROUGH, J.N., BAHULEYAN, K. and CURRY, G.R. (1969). Experimental observations on the origin of the M-echo. *Med. biol. Engng.*, **7**, 465–79.
3.26. WHITE, D.N., CLARK, J.M., WHITE, D.A.W., CAMPBELL, J.K., BAHULEYAN, K., KRAUS, A.S. and BRINKER, R.A. (1971). The deformation of the ultrasonic field in passage across the living and cadaver head. In *Ultrasonographia Medica*, Ed. J. Böck and K. Ossoinig, vol. I, pp. 179–86. Vienna: Verlag Wien. Med. Akad.
3.27. WHITE, D.N. and CURRY, G.R. (1974). Registration errors in midline echoencephalography. *Med. biol. Engng.*, **12**, 712–20.
3.28. WHITE, D.N. and HANNA, L.F. (1974). Automatic midline echoencephalography: 3333 consecutive cases examined with the Automatic Midline Computer. *Neurology*, **24**, 80–93.
3.29. WHITE, D.N. and HUDSON, A.C. (1971). The future of A-mode midline echoencephalography—the development of automated techniques. *Neurology*, **21**, 140–53.
3.30. WHITE, D.N., JENKINS, C.O. and CAMPBELL, J.K. (1970). The compensatory mechanisms for volume changes in the brain. *Proc. 23rd ann. Conf. Engng. Med. Biol.*, Washington, p. 104.
3.31. WHITE, D.N., KRAUS, A.S., CLARK, J.M. and CAMPBELL, J.K. (1969). Interpreter error in echoencephalography. *Neurology*, **19**, 775–84.
3.32. WHITE, D.N. and STEVENSON, R.J. (1975). The causes of transient variations in the magnitude of the systolic pulsations in amplitude recorded from cerebral interfaces: the absence of any relationship with variations in regional blood flow. In *Ultrasound in Medicine*, Ed. D.N. White, vol. 1, pp. 125–63. New York: Plenum Press.

4. Ultrasonic investigations in obstetrics and gynaecology

IAN DONALD

4.1 INTRODUCTION

Looking back to the mid-1950s when work on sonar * first started in Glasgow, it can now be recognized that it was inevitable that the first real breakthrough would come through the medium of gynaecology and obstetrics [4.17, 4.19]. In the first place there was no commercially available apparatus at that time suitable for medical use, nor could engineering firms be expected to take much interest in developing apparatus which might not find sufficiently popular usage to make it commercially viable. Nor at that time was sufficient known about the ultrasonic echo characteristics of tissues *in vivo*. What was needed was a branch of medicine where ultrasonic echoes could be recorded, and the diagnosis confirmed, within a very brief space of time. Gynaecology first [4.22], and subsequently obstetrics, provided just such conditions.

Firstly, abdominal tumours, whether they be gynaecological, or the gravid uterus and its contents, are large and readily palpable and arising out of the pelvis they displaced the ultrasonically impenetrable bowels and commonly come to lie in close proximity to the abdominal wall. Here they are directly accessible to contact scanning with an ultrasonic probe, without interference from bony interfaces. Secondly, most gynaecological tumours come to confirmatory diagnosis at laparotomy and conditions discovered during pregnancy can readily be confirmed in the near future by delivery. There is thus an immediate information feedback.

A successful ultrasonic diagnosis in gynaecology can be triumphantly confirmed while it is still fresh in everyone's minds, and mistakes, however humiliating, encourage very rapid learning. Likewise pregnancy being a condition with a natural tendency to completion within a very few months at most, provides opportunities for self-congratulation and self-criticism.

This kind of rapid information feedback is less commonly available in the case of diseases of liver, heart or spleen, and even the ultimate rostrum of the post-mortem room may be still far off in time, so that the picture may meanwhile alter from the original ultrasonic findings.

The genito-urinary applications of sonar promise to run a close second to gynaecology([4.1]; and see Chapter 8) especially as confirmatory radiological techniques of the most sophisticated sort are nowadays available.

*Professor Donald uses the term '*sonar*' (which is analogous to *radar*) to describe the whole field of ultrasonic diagnosis. One of his reasons for preferring this term is that it distinguishes diagnostic ultrasonic echo sounding, in the mind of the relatively uninformed, from high power ultrasound, the destructive effects of which are already well known. Furthermore it is commended for its brevity, its euphony and the acknowledgment which it accords to its maritime origins, going back to the U-boat campaign of the 1914–18 war.

Ultrasonic echocardiography has made such rapid and astonishing strides in recent years that it may come to outpace in sophistication the present uses of sonar in obstetrics and gynaecology (see Chapter 7).

In reviewing the uses of sonar, the biggest disappointment is in the localization of cerebral tumours—surely the greatest need—because of the technical difficulties provided by the intact skull with its apparently insuperable problems of attenuation and distortion of the ultrasonic beam (see Chapter 3). Indeed sonar finds its great justification in the examination of soft tissue structures, such as are encountered in gynaecology and obstetrics and for which radiology may either be ineffectual, inappropriate or, particularly in the case of pregnancy, potentially harmful.

The initial concern of the clinicians in Glasgow was with the difficult differential diagnosis provided by the grossly enlarged abdomen, distended either with a pelvic tumour or with ascites, or even almost impenetrable degrees of obesity [4.21, 4.22]. It was only in the later parts of the 1950s that observations were extended to obstetrics. From the observations made at that time, a number of general principles [4.22] were enumerated on which to base an inferential diagnosis and, strange as it may seem, these principles appear to have stood the test of time.

4.2. GENERAL PRINCIPLES OF DIAGNOSIS

Bearing in mind the limitations of two-dimensional scanning, including the fact that tissue interfaces may present in a plane in a third dimension which is not normal to the incident ultrasonic beam, it is seldom wise to make a diagnosis on the basis of any one scan. It may be necessary to take a large number of cuts both longitudinal, at different distances from the midline, and in transverse section, at different levels and angles of tilt. Occasionally for specialized information, such as in the search for both heads simultaneously in diagnosing twins, an oblique scan is necessary.

These multiple scans, if photographed in every instance, are very wasteful in time and in photographic materials. Therefore, in adopting a search technique it is worthwhile to have a cathode ray tube with a medium persistence phosphor (1−2 s at most), so that the picture fades rapidly. This prevents confusion from overwriting, and enables the search to be carried out under direct vision. Alternatively, a storage display with rapid erase facilities may enable the desired view to be obtained. Unfortunately, direct view storage tubes have relatively poor dynamic range and resolution. In either case, Polaroid* photography may be used to make permanent records of selected scans.

Compound scanning is normally employed, but with the improved sensitivity of more modern scanners, there is a tendency to use less compounding in order to obtain improved resolution. Coupling is achieved with a liberal film of olive or arachis oil smeared on the patient's skin. A common mistake is not to use enough of the coupling medium.

Because of the need to find the correct plane to obtain the best pictures, the scanning probe and the arms on which it is mounted should be easily manoeuv-

*Registered trademark of Polaroid Corporation, Cambridge, MA 02139, USA.

rable. A good longitudinal scan is worth about half a dozen transverse scans and yet many machines on the market are clumsy in converting from longitudinal to transverse views and *vice versa*. Versatility of operation is particularly important, not only to secure good results but also to save time and get through the number of cases required. In Glasgow it is common to undertake a dozen or more in a day and normally four examinations are made in an hour, including all documentation. Speed of operation is particularly important in patients in late pregnancy, because many do not tolerate lying on their backs for long periods of time and begin to feel sick and dizzy from the supine hypotensive syndrome, which is due to inferior vena caval compression by the weight of the gravid uterus. If this happens, either the examination must be called off and the patient turned onto her side, or a few extra minutes can be won by raising the patient's outstretched legs high in the air on the shoulders of an assistant to improve the venous return to the heart.

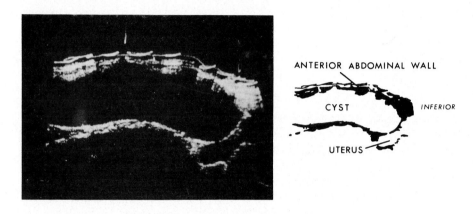

Fig. 4.1 Very large ovarian cyst in longitudinal section (at 5 MHz), pressing upon a retroverted uterus.

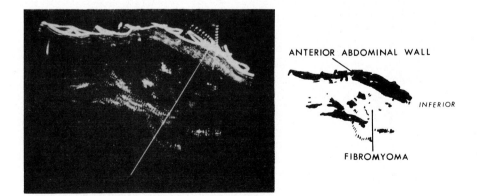

Fig. 4.2 Fibromyoma in longitudinal section (at 1·5 MHz), with some areas of calcification. In comparison with Fig. 4.1, note the relative lack of transonicity.

In interpreting ultrasonic information, the frequency employed is an important consideration. The higher the frequency, the less the penetration by ultrasound, and *vice versa*. Therefore, a solid tumour is harder to 'see through', or in other words is less 'transonic' then a cystic mass. By using a lower frequency, for example, 1·5 MHz instead of 2·5 MHz (which is the standard frequency in Glasgow), it should usually be possible to outline the posterior, deeper surface of fairly dense tumours such as fibromyomas of the uterus. Even at this frequency, however, this is almost impossible in the case of a very dense fibroma of ovary. A fluid-containing structure, on the other hand, offers minimal attenuation to the passage of the ultrasonic beam, therefore its outline may be very easily mapped out even at frequencies as high as 5 MHz. This effect is illustrated* in Figs. 4.1

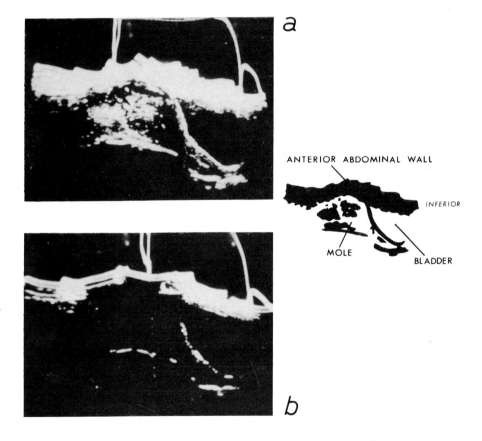

Fig. 4.3 Hydatidiform mole in longitudinal section (at 5 MHz). Both scans show the same scan plane, but (*a*) was made with a system sensitivity of 10 dB greater than for (*b*). Note that the lower sensitivity extinguished the speckled appearance of the mole, but not the posterior uterine wall.

*The ultrasonograms which illustrate this Chapter were all made with the *'Diasonograph'* apparatus (Nuclear Enterprises Ltd., Edinburgh, E11 4EY, UK), using models NE 4102, and, for gray scale pictures, NE 4104. This instrument is a manually operated contact scanner (see Section 2.1.*e*).

and 4.2. As is pointed out in Chapters 1 and 2, the strengths of the echoes which are received depend upon the differences in the characteristic impedances of the tissues on either side of the reflecting interfaces, and these may be different for different tissues. In this respect the differences between placental tissue, uterine wall and certain fetal structures may be only marginal, and therefore very accurate and careful sensitivity settings are necessary.

This explains why success was not immediate in ultrasonic placentography. In fact it was first found that hydatidiform mole is visible as a speckled mass at a sensitivity about 15 dB higher than that at which it becomes almost invisible (returning no intrauterine echoes) although the deeper surface of the far uterine wall remains outlined in full [4.21, 4.30]. This is illustrated in Fig. 4.3.

It was from recognizing how to identify hydatidiform mole that the method was evolved of differentiating between placental tissue and liquor amnii by increasing the sensitivity so that placental echoes showed up as speckles which are not present in the case of clear liquor [4.20]. Sensitivity settings have to be individual since the range of transonicity varies from patient to patient and depends on the thickness of the skin and the abdominal wall.

The pelvic viscera (for example the normal, non-pregnant uterus), if not sufficiently enlarged to be palpable above the level of the symphysis pubis, cannot be displayed by sonar examination carried out through the anterior abdominal wall because intervening bowel is impenetrable. Bowel is impenetrable because it always contains gas, which almost totally reflects a diagnostic ultrasonic beam. By allowing the patient's bladder to fill with urine, however, the intestine is displaced out of the way. The bladder thus provides a built-in 'viewing tank' through which to examine the immediately subjacent uterus and its contents and, unfortunately with less certainty, the uterine appendages [4.9]. Since this discovery it has been possible to examine the human embryo at its earliest growth from the fifth or sixth week of amenorrhoea onwards [4.10, 4.13].

When examining a mass or structure which is lying behind bowel, a satisfactory ultrasonogram can only be obtained either by displacing the bowel with the full bladder, or by approaching it from a different part of the body. Normal

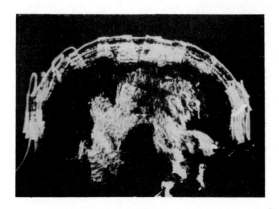
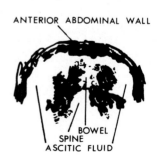

ANTERIOR ABDOMINAL WALL

BOWEL
SPINE
ASCITIC FLUID

Fig. 4.4 Ascites due to carcinomatosis peritonei. Transverse section at 2·5 MHz.

kidneys can thus be examined through the patient's back in the prone position, even in the absence of any enlargement. Examination of the liver, especially if not clinically enlarged, likewise presents difficulties which often require some ingenuity to circumvent (see Chapter 6). Even so present day restrictions to two-dimensional scanning may make the inspection of the liver substance incomplete.

The very fact that gas-containing bowel presents such strong reflecting interfaces can, however, be made use of in examining cases of ascites. If the fluid in the peritoneal cavity is truly free, and not loculated, and if the bowel is consequently free to float up into the centre of the abdomen, as usually occurs with the patient in the dorsal positon, the fluid can be seen to be wholly congregated within the flanks, as shown in Fig. 4.4; whereas if there is malignant infiltration involving intestine, omentum and other viscera, the picture becomes much more irregular and bizarre. This is a useful diagnostic point and provides a picture which is pathognomonic of, for example, malignant ascites due to peritoneal carcinomatosis.

It is a pity that, at present, it is impossible to differentiate between one kind of fluid and another, for example, between pus, blood, urine or any other biological fluid. It may be appreciated that ultrasonic diagnosis is by no means necessarily pictorial, but often depends upon inference, for example, from the way in which a mass is displaced or the clarity of its outline, or its relationship to other structures and so forth. Sonar has widened the scope of diagnosis but has certainly not made it any easier.

4.3 THE DOPPLER EFFECT

A somewhat different application of ultrasonic echo sounding is to be found in the use of the Doppler effect. By this means any accessible structure which pulsates or moves can be studied. A reflecting interface, by its movement, alters the apparent frequency of the returning echo received, and this alteration in frequency can be processed in a number of ways. In obstetrics and gynaecology, the obvious target of interest is the fetal heart, although blood vessels with an active pulsing circulation can also provide ultrasonic Doppler shift signals [4.2, 4.28]. In the case of the fetal heart, alterations in rate from beat to beat can be instantly computed. Doppler shift signals from the fetal heart can be picked up occasionally at 10 weeks, often at 11 weeks, and with increasing certainty from 13 weeks onwards. They provide incontrovertible proof of continuing intrauterine fetal life.

Ordinary clinical methods of assessing changes in fetal heart rate, which are an important index of fetal wellbeing, are much handicapped during the height of a powerful uterine contraction in labour, since direct auscultation at such a time becomes difficult or impossible. Fetal electrocardiography is nowadays commonly employed to monitor fetal heart rate in labour, but this requires the application of an electrode to the presenting part, and is consequently only available after the membranes have ruptured. Before the membranes have ruptured, ultrasonic Doppler examination is the only worthwhile method of monitoring the fetal heart, since it registers primarily the movement of the pulsating heart, and is not greatly influenced by extraneous signals. All previous techniques of phonocardiography, however expensive, have by now been discarded because of the frustrating artifacts to which they were liable.

4.4 APPLICATIONS OF SONAR

In this section, some examples are given of the different clinical conditions which can be profitably examined by sonar. The subject has also been reviewed elsewhere [4.14, 4.18]. The various indications for sonar investigation are listed in Table 4.1.

Table 4.1. Indications in obstetrics for investigations by sonar.

Early pregnancy	Middle and late pregnancy	Puerperium
Early gestation sac	Fetal growth rate	Retained products
Implantation	Maturity	Involution
Growth rate	Twins	Caesarean section scars
Blighted ovum	Associated tumours	Haematoma
Placental differentiation	Hydramnios	Associated tumours
Maturity	Placental localization	
Early diagnosis of twins	Placental development	
Investigation of abortion	Rh placental changes	
Retained products of	Caesarean section scar	
conception	integrity	
Hydatidiform mole	Renal complications	
Associated pelvic tumours		
Ectopic pregnancy		
Renal complications		

4.4.a. Early pregnancy

The full bladder technique, as mentioned in Section 4.2, makes this a particularly rewarding field. It is possible to see a gestation sac within the uterus and its level of nidation, in many cases from the fifth week of pregnancy (menstrual age) onwards, and if it cannot be found by the sixth week there begins to be doubt whether the patient is pregnant at all. Furthermore the rate of growth of the gestation sac is now well known, and gives a good indication of the viability of the pregnancy [4.13].

It should always be possible, whenever the appearance of a gestation sac is obtained by longitudinal scanning, to be able also to reveal it by transverse scanning. This is illustrated in Fig. 4.5.

Twins demonstrate two gestation sacs. The famous Hanson quintuplets were diagnosed at the ninth week of amenorrhoea using this technique which was altogether a remarkable feat [4.5]. In Glasgow, the existence of twin gestation sacs has been recognized at seven and a half weeks of amenorrhoea [4.12]. Sometimes the diagnosis of pregnancy can be established before the urine tests themselves are positive.

It is now recognized that early pregnancy failure as a form of human biological wastage is very common: in fact it is likely that 25 per cent would not be an

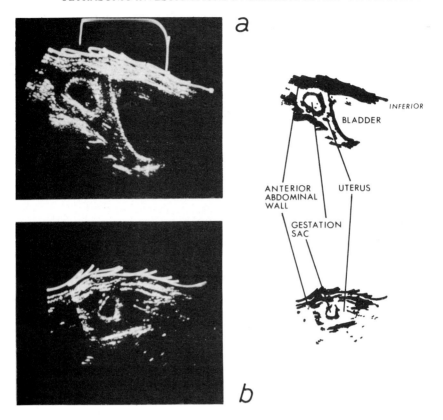

Fig. 4.5 Seven to eight week gestation, showing the gestation sac in (a) longitudinal section, and (b) transverse section. Frequency = 2·5 MHz.

overestimate. It is difficult to give a true incidence since many cases of early pregnancy failure are not reported, but in a series [4.34] of 425 consecutive patients examined by sonar in the first half of pregnancy, no less than 176 ultimately aborted. This is almost certainly an exagerration of the true figure of wastage, since it is necessary to take into account the reasons for which these patients were referred for ultrasonic examination in the first place, but the phenomenon of ovum-blighting has been recognised for many years and the introduction of sonar has now made the diagnosis of this condition possible. To many unfortunate women the phenomenon of recurrent abortion in early pregnancy is a particularly discouraging matter. Many are not aware that they are ever pregnant since after a brief period of amenorrhoea they pass whatever is inside the uterus as what is apparently a heavy menstrual loss. Therefore, it is unusual to obtain a specimen for proper pathological examination unless the patient herself has been alerted to the possibility in advance.

In the search to establish the diagnosis of blighted ovum by sonar, material has been picked from 141 cases of bleeding in the first trimester of pregnancy, and correlated with the findings obtained at the first and subsequent ultrasonic examinations [4.23]. In 66 patients who aborted, the suggestion of a blighted ovum had given characteristic ultrasonic appearances in no less than 57, whereas in 10 of the 75 patients in whom pregnancy continued, the ultrasonic appearance was abnormal on at least one occasion.

Many varieties of early pregnancy failure are now recognized, and the ultrasonic feature of blighted ovum have been listed as follows:

(i) An absence of fetal echoes within the gestation sac. (It should be possible to find fetal echoes within such a sac occasionally from the fifth week of amenorrhoea, commonly at the sixth week, and with certainty by the seventh week.) This condition is called 'anembryonic'. When the products of conception are finally obtained, only portions of sac and fragments of unrecognizable embryonic remnants can be found.

(ii) A loss of definition of the gestation sac. This may be accompanied by the appearance of speckling and occasionally a break in the contour of the sac giving a sort of C-shape appearance.

(iii) A gestation sac which is unquestionably small for dates and on re-examination a week later no appreciable growth would appear to have occurred. Occasionally there may even be shrinkage of the sac volume.

(iv) A low position sac within the uterus. This often, though not invariably, indicates a poor prognosis. In some of these cases, it may be that the beginning of the abortion process itself is being observed.

In Glasgow, the term 'blighted ovum' is limited to the anembryonic sac in which no fetal parts can be demonstrated, either by sonar or subsequently on examination of the aborted products of conception, and the term 'missed abortion' is used when a fetus can be seen, and measured by sonar, but in which no fetal heart movements can at any time be detected. A far smaller group of 'live abortions' is recognized if fetal heart movements can be demonstrated by sonar within a few days before spontaneous abortion, or if there are no signs of maceration, and the size of the fetus is compatible with the period of amenorrhoea [4.34].

Three techniques may be relied upon as an objective measure for recognising the pregnancy that is doomed from the first, as compared with one which has a good prognosis. The most important of these is the detection of fetal heart movements by time-position scanning [4.32].

The demonstration of fetal heart movement in very early pregnancy depends upon first locating the fetal mass, usually lying by gravity towards the posterior wall of the gestation sac, and then scanning slowly and carefully through this mass, searching for signs of fetal heart pulsation. This is recognized first of all on an A-scan on which the movement of the fetal heart is represented by the appropriate echo moving from left to right and vice versa. The search can be coned down further by the use of superimposed electronic cursors. The apparatus is then switched to the time-position mode to produce a recording such as that shown in Fig. 4.6. The rate, and even the extent of movement can be measured with great accuracy. The fetal heart commonly has a rate between 160–180 min^{-1} at this time and no further source of pulsation within the human body could produce such a picture. This is proof positive of fetal life, and if it cannot be

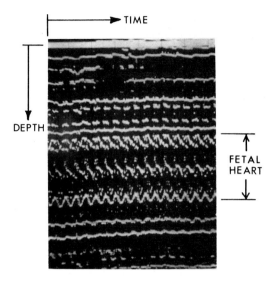

Fig. 4.6 Fetal heart demonstrated by time-position scanning at ten weeks gestation (menstrual age).

obtained by the seventh week of amenorrhoea and certainly by the eighth week of amenorrhoea there is doubt about the existence of a living and surviving pregnancy. Since the fetus can be so easily found, if present, within a gestation sac, the technique of measuring the crown-rump length was developed, and this distance has been related to maturity [4.33, 4.35]. Within the first 10 or 12 weeks of pregnancy, an estimate of maturity to within half a week is obtainable, with practice, and this information may be of the greatest value later on. The prior use of the contraceptive pill, and any history of menstrual irregularity, produces a common doubt as to the real maturity of a given pregnancy. Sonar at this early stage can resolve it.

Finally, the volume of the gestation sac itself has been found to be of great value in assessing the prognosis for a given pregnancy. It should be possible to detect, not only the fetus, but fetal heart movements as well, in any gestation sac with a volume of 2 ml or more [4.32, 4.34]; and all pregnancies with a gestation sac volume of less than 5 ml more than double that volume within the course of one week. The volume can be calculated by taking maximum diameter scans in more than one plane. The absence of fetal echoes in a gestation sac, with a volume of more than 2·5 ml, makes the diagnosis of anembryonic blighted ovum practically certain. Nevertheless, allowing for possible mistaken dates, a sac smaller than 2·5 ml might require re-examination in a week's time to see if there is any increase. Using these criteria it has now become the practice to diagnose blighted ovum with confidence, and to terminate the pregnancy forthwith. On no occasion in Glasgow has a firm diagnosis of this condition been made which was subsequently shown to be normal.

When bleeding occurs in early pregnancy, or in a woman with a bad obstetric history, the differential diagnosis is often difficult, especially if the urine tests are positive. Here sonar can be of enormous value since it can distinguish definitely

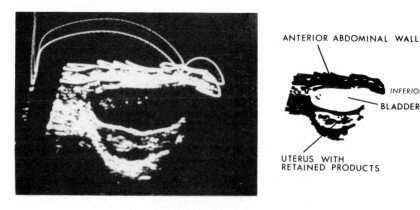

ANTERIOR ABDOMINAL WALL

INFERIOR
BLADDER

UTERUS WITH
RETAINED PRODUCTS

Fig. 4.7 Retained products of conception resulting from incomplete abortion. Longitudinal section at 2·5 MHz.

between a continuing pregnancy and one which is doomed. It can also differentiate between an incomplete abortion, as shown in Fig. 4.7, and an abortion which is only threatened and worth struggling to salve.

Other differential diagnoses of bleeding from the uterine cavity in early pregnancy can also be resolved by sonar, for example, when due to hydatidiform mole, and in suspected ectopic pregnancy where the unequivocal finding of an intrauterine gestation sac rules out the likelihood of such a diagnosis. The ultrasonic findings in cases of ectopic pregnancy, however, are very variable and often difficult to interpret. As might be expected, they depend on whether or not the Fallopian tube has actually ruptured; on the amount of pelvic haematocele, and on the degree of haemoperitoneum. Nevertheless, in all subacute cases of suspected ectopic pregnancy, an ultrasonic examination is worthwhile if only to exclude a normal intrauterine pregnancy with a threat to abort, or to indicate the need for laparoscopy to confirm the diagnosis.

It is interesting to watch the differentiation of the chorion frondosum from the chorion laevi in the first appearances of the placenta. The process can be observed starting as early as the eighth or ninth week of amenorrhoea, and it seems that a placenta which appears to be differentiating in the upper uterine segment, even at this stage, does not later present as a case of placenta praevia. On the other hand, the placenta may appear to be developing over the lower uterine segment and this alerts to the possibility of bleeding in the near future, or the later development of placenta praevia. Fortunately, in many of these cases the placenta appears actively to migrate and as the lower uterine segment in later pregnancy differentiates, so may an apparently unfavourable placenta come to occupy a less dangerous position within the uterus [4.29].

4.4.b. Accurate assessment of maturity in the first half of pregnancy
This has now become a vitally important matter with the increasing use of amniocentesis, and with the growing science of diagnosing fetal abnormality at a stage early enough to permit termination. The levels of alphafetoprotein in the liquor amnii very markedly in accordance with maturity, which must always be

taken into account in assessing their significance. The specimens are obtained by amniocentesis which, in itself, demands localization of the placenta by sonar, in order to avoid damage to the placenta by the exploring needle, and with the danger of possible iso-immunization of the mother in susceptible cases. Alpha-fetoprotein levels are significantly raised in congenital neural tube defects of the fetus, but for the results to be meaningful the maturity of the fetus must be known. The patient's history is not sufficiently reliable. If a sonar examination has been undertaken in very early pregnancy there is no doubt, but even between the twelfth and the twentieth week of pregnancy the size of the head is so closely related to maturity, and in fact grows so rapidly, that all doubt should be resolved. What is even more important in undertaking amniocentesis in cases of suspected neural tube defect, is to exclude the presence of twins, which can only be done at this stage by sonar since x-radiology is not applicable.

In Glasgow, all pregnant women are screened in early pregnancy by estimating the serum alphafetoprotein. The serum levels of this substance are very markedly affected by the degree of maturity, which must be absolutely known before they can be accepted as meaningful. They provide an indication for amniocentesis, the interpretation of which depends, though to a less critical extent, upon the estimate of maturity.

4.4.c. Middle and late pregnancy

The vault of the fetal skull is the easiest part to identify in an ultrasonic scan since the bones show up very well. If properly scanned in the appropriate plane, it appears as an almost complete circle. In certain views this can be confused with the fetal thorax but this mistake can be avoided by searching for the midline structures of the fetal brain usually ascribed to the falx cerebri. No such structure is to be found within the apparently circular section of the fetal thorax. An additional precaution is to identify the fetal head with certainty in more than one scan plane, but even better is the demonstration of the fetal heart within the structure in question. The presence of a pulsating fetal heart in this situation positively identifies the structure as a thorax and not, for example, as a second fetal head as might be expected in twins [4.16].

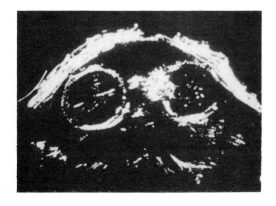
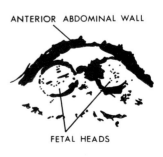

Fig. 4.8 Twin heads at 25 weeks gestation. Transverse section at 2·5 MHz.

Since finding the head is so easy, the diagnosis of presentation can be settled more quickly than by any other non-clinical method. This is particularly useful in difficult cases of suspected breech presentation and should unhesitatingly be used before resorting to external cephalic version in all but the most obvious cases. Obesity and gross distension from hydramnios provide no difficulties to a proper sonar examination.

The diagnosis of twins is conveniently made by identifying two separate heads at separate levels. Having ascertained that each structure is a fetal head, an endeavour should then be made to obtain a picture of both simultaneously in one appropriately oblique scan. This often requires quite refined adjustment of the position of the scan plane, as illustrated in Fig. 4.8.

4.4.d. Diagnosis of fetal abnormality

The prenatal diagnosis of fetal abnormality is rapidly opening up almost as a subject in its own right [4.26]. Apart from assisting the correct performance of amniocentesis, sonar is beginning to show promise as a method of identifying at least certain cases of structural defect, particularly of head and spine. The matter is all the more important since x-radiology is useless before the eighteenth week and often later due to inadequate calcification of the fetal skeleton.

Anencephaly can be diagnosed even in the first half of pregnancy and should always be sought in all cases of hydramnios which, in itself, produces characteristic appearances of black spaces with white, blob-like, echoes [4.36]. If a fetal head cannot be seen and measured at the sixteenth week of pregnancy, it is justifiable to question whether the baby in fact has one. A presumptive diagnosis of anencephaly can then be confirmed by amniocentesis and estimation of alphafetoprotein. There should be fewer and fewer tragedies of the late discovery of anencephaly in a woman who has already become far advanced in pregnancy and occasionally dangerously postmature.

Spinal defects are more difficult to recognise because of the problem of following a curving structure, such as fetal spine, in one two-dimensional plane [4.6].

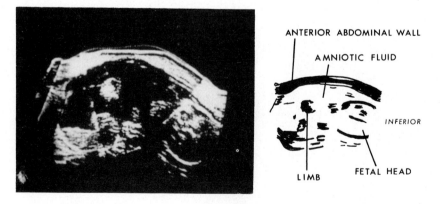

Fig. 4.9 Hydramnios. Note blob-like echoes. Posterior placenta and engaged head on right side of picture.

4.4.e. Large-for-dates pregnancy

A common reason for referral for ultrasonic examination is the suggestion that the patient is much larger than is consistent with her dates. Sonar resolves the problem very readily, and distinguishes such causes as mistaken dates, multiple pregnancy, hydramnios, and associated and hitherto unsuspected pelvic tumours (see Figs. 4.9, 4.16 and 4.17).

Hydrocephalus, on the other hand, commonly does not reveal itself until the second half of pregnancy when it can be recognized as an abnormally large head; in fact any biparietal diameter exceeding 110 mm must raise this suspicion and call for confirmatory radiology.

4.5. BIPARIETAL CEPHALOMETRY

Since the head is easy to find, it is also fairly easy to measure it. The measurement of greatest clinical usefulness and the only one of any constancy in the fetus is the biparietal diameter. The rationale of the original technique is the fact that echoes

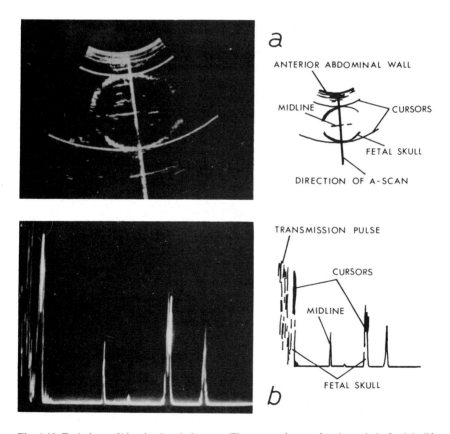

Fig. 4.10 Technique of biparietal cephalometry. The appropriate section through the fetal skull is first identified using the two-dimensional B-scope, as shown in (a). The cursors of the electronic caliper are set to coincide with the parietal bones. The display is then presented on the A-scope, as shown in (b). Finally, the cursors are adjusted more exactly, and the biparietal diameter is read off from the calibrated control. Frequency = 2·5 MHz.

of comparable magnitude, from the parietal bones on each side, are only recorded on A-scan when the ultrasonic beam traverses the head through a true diameter and not a chord [4.21]. Confusion with the only other true diameter at right angles (the occipito-frontal diameter) is fortunately obviated, firstly by the fact that this diameter is usually incaccesible because the head engages in the brim of the pelvis in the transverse diameter, and secondly because it is so much larger that the mistake is not likely to be made. Finally the midline echo, believed due to the falx, should always be sought at the same time. Measurement of the biparietal diameter must be very accurate to be of much clinical use.

The first serial measurements of biparietal growth in successive patients were made in Glasgow [4.38, 4.39]. Since then, the technique has been enormously improved and refined by first identifying the head on a two-dimensional scan to show the midline echo, and then by carefully centering the beam to pass through the widest diameter of the head with the midline exactly at right angles. The distance between the two parietal bones is measured on A-scan. The procedure is illustrated in Fig. 4.10 [4.3]. Measurement from a graticule on the screen of the cathode ray tube is considered to be totally inadequate, and so electronically generated cursors are superimposed to brighten the trace at positions coinciding with the leading edges of the appropriate echoes. The distance between the cursors should be directly calibrated on the manipulating dials taking into account the velocity of sound through fetal brain. This is assumed to be 1600 m s^{-1}, and the accuracy aimed at is 0.5 mm^*. Biparietal cephalometry makes it possible to study the progressive growth of the fetal head and to relate this to certain conditions in pregnancy which might interfere with that growth (for example dysmaturity, maternal hypertension, diabetes and renal disease) [4.4, 4.38, 4.39]. The measurement of the biparietal diameter is not only useful for the determination of maturity (in this respect it is a great improvement on other methods, especially between the twentieth and thirtieth weeks of pregnancy [4.4]), but it may indicate a slackening rate of fetal growth with the implied threat of placental subnutrition, or, as it is fashionably called, 'placental insufficiency', or even of intrauterine death. An even more precise method of estimating fetal growth can be achieved by simultaneously employing ultrasonic thoracometry, which helps to give a better idea of the fetal weight than cephalometry alone, and a very wide experience has now been accumulated in this combined technique [4.7, 4.25, 4.27].

This technique of monitoring intrauterine wellbeing should be used in all cases of previous history of dysmaturity, and in maternal conditions threatening to the fetus, and when the baby appears clinically small-for-dates. The opinion so obtained is further reinforced by simultaneous oestriol excretion studies. In Glasgow, a double reference chart (Fig. 4.11) is employed; this shows the Campbell normal fetal biparietal growth rate and the Coyle oestriol excretion chart on the same sheet [4.8, 4.12]. In this way complementary evidence indicates failures in fetal growth. When there is an appreciable discrepancy between fetal head growth and maternal oestriol excretion rates a possible explanation should be sought, bearing in mind even the possibility of some major abnormality, in

---

*Many investigators use a velocity of 1580 m s^{-1}, and few aim to achieve an accuracy of better than 1 mm—editor.

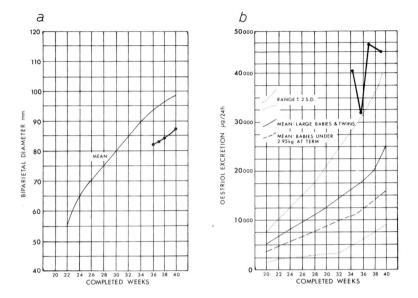

Fig. 4.11 Charts showing normal values of (a) biparietal diameter, and (b) oestriol excretion. The example shows measurements made for a microcephalic fetus, with correspondingly high oestriol excretion rates.

which case the diagnosis must finally rest on the characteristic radiological findings.

Biparietal cephalometry is not only the most commonly required type of ultrasonic examination in obstetrics but it is also one of the most difficult, and there are many pitfalls for the inexperienced [4.15]. The proper finding and orientation of the midline structures is essential, and the best procedure is first to superimpose the cursors on the parietal eminences on the B-scan, using the maximum magnification available, in preparation for final adjustment on the A-scan.

4.6 PLACENTOGRAPHY

The first report of successful placentography by sonar came from the United States [4.24], and this was soon followed by a similar report from Glasgow [4.20]. The principles are illustrated in Fig. 4.12.

Wherever this service is available, sonar is generally accepted as the preferred special technique for localizing the placenta. It has many advantages, quite apart from its high reliability rate (even in the early Glasgow series this was just over 94 per cent). It can be undertaken at any hour of day or night, and the seriously ill patient does not have to be moved from her bed although examination on a couch is always easier. No radioactive isotopes have to be dispensed, nor is any special radiological technique required. Furthermore, the examination can be repeated as often as desired without known hazard to the patient or to her fetus. Perhaps an even more useful feature is that the earlier in pregnancy the localization is carried out, the easier it is, as shown in Fig. 4.13.

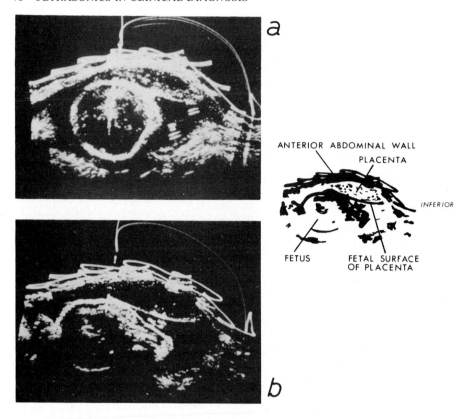

Fig. 4.12 Placentography. Longitudinal sections at 2·5 MHz. Note the fetal surface of the placenta. Both scans show the same scan plane, but (a) was made with a system sensitivity of 10 dB greater than for (b). Note that the lower sensitivity extinguishes the speckled appearance of the placenta: this test helps in the distinction from liquor amnii.

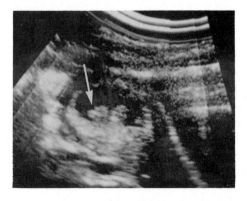

Fig. 4.13 Nine weeks gestation sac (menstrual age) showing fetus lying on posteriorly situated placenta which is differentiating and beginning to develop in the upper uterine segment (arrow). Oblique view. Gray-scale imaging technique.

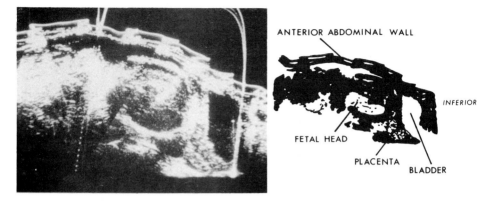

Fig. 4.14 Major degree of placenta praevia. Longitudinal section at 2·5 MHz. The placenta comes down from the anterior and lies over the internal os of the cervix behind the partially filled bladder.

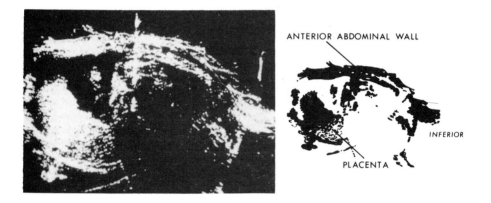

Fig. 4.15 Rhesus placenta of 33 weeks gestation. Longitudinal section at 2·5 MHz. The baby required two exchange transfusions.

The phenomenon of 'placental migration' has been mentioned already. This is the case in which the placenta is seen at an earlier stage in pregnancy to be situated low, and even in the praevia position and yet, as pregnancy advances, and the lower uterine segment 'takes up', the situation is seen to improve. The reverse phenomenon has not been seen, so that a placenta at an earlier stage of pregnancy, once localized wholly in the upper uterine segment, can, with confidence, not be suspected of adopting a later praevia position.

Ultrasonic placentography is indicated in all cases of antepartum haemorrhage, where there is an unstable lie of the fetus, whether or not haemorrhage has occurred, and always before amniocentesis.

There are certain pitfalls of which to be aware in interpreting placentograms. It is always worth searching for the white line which reveals the fetal surface of the placenta. This is most likely to be found if the ultrasonic beam is perpendicular to that surface and this may require a certain amount of adjustment of the scan plane.

The opacity or otherwise of the placental echo pattern depends upon many things, for example, on the amount of liquor in the uterus and whether or not the main mass of the fetal trunk is putting it partly into 'shadow'. The presence of the placenta may, in fact should be, confirmed by altering the sensitivity by 10 − 15 dB, so as to show both the space occupied by the presumed placenta and, at the higher sensitivity, the same area filled with speckles. It is always useful to have some urine in the patient's bladder, about 100 ml, in order to reveal the level of the lower segment of the uterus when searching for placenta praevia. An example of this is shown in Fig. 4.14.

The physical properties of the placenta in various diseases are also of interest, although their study by ultrasound is still not far advanced. It has already been noticed, however, that cases of serious rhesus iso-immunization show the sonar appearances of a thick, opaque placenta [4.16]: this is illustrated in Fig. 4.15.

The actual texture of the placenta, especially bearing in mind such matters as diffuse infarction, requires a more refined and up-to-date technique such as gray scale echography.

4.7. HYDATIDIFORM MOLE

Nowadays, sonar undoubtedly provides the quickest and most certain method of diagnosing this very dangerous condition, by employing the general principle that speckles are revealed by increasing the sensitivity setting, as described in Section 4.2. This speckled appearance can be suppressed by reducing the sensitivity of the apparatus by 10 − 15 dB, whereas fetal echoes quite definitely cannot. This method of examination is far more satisfactory and reliable than biochemical estimations of gonadotrophin levels, and may save the patient weeks of unnecessary bleeding, uncertainty, toxaemia and the ever-present danger of subsequent malignant change. There is a serious pitfall: this is to mistake a degenerate fibromyoma for a hydatidiform mole [4.11]. In order to avoid this possibility, the diagnosis should be confirmed at a frequency of 5 MHz as well as at the standard 2·5 MHz. It is important always to recognize that a hydatidiform mole, because of its vascularity, is highly transonic and even though the speckles may be suppressed by reducing the gain the view of the posterior wall of the uterus should always be seen (see Fig. 4.3).

4.8. PELVIC TUMOURS ASSOCIATED WITH PREGNANCY

The clinical problem of the abdomen which is larger than the menstrual dates would suggest has already been mentioned. Commonly associated pelvic tumours with pregnancy are ovarian cysts and fibromyomata. The distinction is extremely important since ovarian cysts demand laparotomy, whereas fibromyomata are best managed by conservative treatment. Therefore the distinction between the two may make all the difference not only in the treatment but to the patient's very life, to say nothing of the outcome of the pregnancy. A fibromyoma in pregnancy, however, is more transonic than in the non-pregnant state, and allowance has to be made for this. This is where a 5 MHz probe is particularly useful, since an ovarian cyst is readily transonic even at this high frequency. Figs. 4.16 and 4.17 illustrate these points.

A tumour deep within the pelvis may prevent the presenting part from engaging and may obstruct labour. Here too, sonar readily demonstrates its nature.

4.9. CAESAREAN SECTION SCARS

The integrity or otherwise of a Caesarean section scar is important not only in the woman previously delivered by this means and now approaching term in a second pregnancy, but also in the post-operative case where the puerperium is apparently abnormal. Nowadays most scars in the lower uterine segment are transverse and therefore it is necessary to take a large number of serial longitudinal scans. Commonly the scar region can be recognized through a full bladder by a puckered area on the scan, although a wellhealed scar may be hard

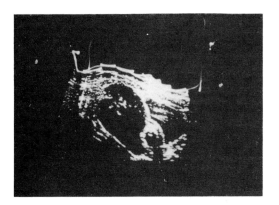
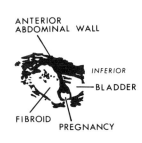

Fig. 4.16 Large degenerate fibroid above an 8–9 week pregnancy, lying behind a semi-filled bladder. Longitudinal section at 2·5 MHz. (*Courtesy*: Patricia Morley.)

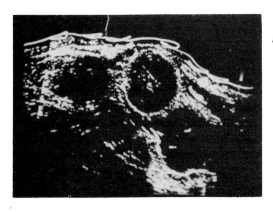
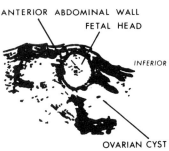

Fig. 4.17 Large ovarian cyst below a fetal head at 36 weeks gestation. Longitudinal section at 2·5 MHz. Elective Caesarian section.

to identify [4.16]. It is not yet possible to diagnose antepartum scar dehiscence with confidence, but signs of puckering and distortion are suspicious. An example is shown in Fig. 4.18. This naturally encourages extra caution in the supervision of a subsequent labour.

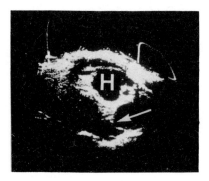

Fig. 4.18 Caesarean section scar dehisced (arrow) with formation of large haematoma (H).

A stormy convalescence following Caesarean section is now recognised as commonly being due either to wound separation, or to faulty haemostasis so that a haematoma collects in the region of the scar and behind the bladder. Formerly these cases were regarded as 'septic'. Sonar can reveal the presence of often a sizeable haematoma. The importance of this observation is that it indicates the need for later hysterosalpingography and the full assessment of the ability of the uterus to withstand a subsequent pregnancy and labour.

4.10. RENAL COMPLICATIONS OF PREGNANCY

Pyelography is generally regarded as being undesirable in pregnancy because of the ionizing radiation which is involved. Fortunately the kidneys are readily accessible to ultrasonic examination especially through the patient's back using the prone position which can be quite comfortably tolerated up to the twenty-sixth week of pregnancy, as described in Chapter 8. Normal cases can easily be distinguished from certain common causes of recurrent urinary infection in pregnancy or in cases of unexplained pyrexia. Hydronephrosis is very readily seen both in longitudinal and transverse sections and, as shown in Fig. 4.19, appears in the form of a 'C' with the open part facing medially. Cases of massive hydronephrosis can be examined more readily with a patient in the dorsal position. Likewise non-functioning kidneys can be examined, and also cases of polycystic disease.

4.11. GYNAECOLOGICAL TUMOURS

The sonar examination of gynaecological tumours should be part of the routine pre-operative work-up. Much useful information may be obtained pre-operatively, and some unpleasant surprises may be avoided in the operating theatre. Multilocular cysts such as pseudomucinous cystadenomata may show a

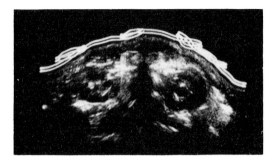 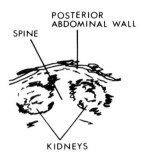

Fig. 4.19 Bilateral hydronephrosis at 21 weeks gestation. Patient in prone position.

number of echoes from the partitions between the loculi and yet the cyst may be simple. Malignant tumours may sometimes look fairly innocent by sonar, and it would be a mistake to try to assess by conventional methods whether or not a tumour is malignant from its ultrasonic appearances. Nevertheless, as a general rule, the more complex a tumour and the echo pattern within it, the more likely is it to be malignant. This is illustrated in Fig. 4.20. Associated ascites is always an important observation, especially as its presence suggests malignancy.

It is important when assessing ascites to delineate the lower border of the liver, since the relatively clear area of a healthy liver may be misinterpreted as ascitic fluid. Therefore, longitudinal scans should be taken not only in the midline but also at about 50 mm to the right and along the lower border of the costal margins, especially when dealing with suspected hepatomegaly or splenomegaly.

The finding of the true size of an ovarian tumour may well determine the type of incision employed at laparotomy, since it is usual practice to endeavour to remove such tumours intact without rupture. This may contraindicate the use of Pfannenstiel incision.

Grossly obese patients may have so protuberant an abdomen that it may be hard to exclude the possibility of an underlying pelvic tumour which cannot be

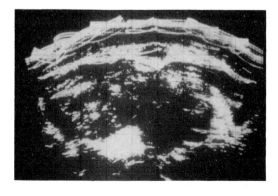 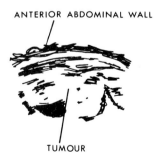

Fig. 4.20 Large ovarian tumour in transverse section. Complex echo pattern indicates malignant nature. Confirmed at laparotomy.

palpated because of the sheer thickness of the abdominal wall. There is no difficulty in penetrating fat with ultrasound, and the existence of such a tumour can be confirmed or excluded very simply.

Pulsation in an abdominal tumour is easily demonstrated by sonar, especially if a time-position recording is made of the pulsating walls [4.21]. Only the anterior wall of an aneurysm pulsates, since the back of the aneurysm is pressed against the unyielding vertebral column; but, for example, a cyst of the pancreas or the lesser sac lying in front of the aorta demonstrates pulsation in both its anterior and posterior walls.

Retroperitoneal tumours, especially deep within the pelvis, are not very satisfactory objects for study by sonar, because of overlying bowel when viewed from in front, and the attenuation in the bony sacrum from behind. Bowel tumours, however, though palpable clinically, may declare their non-gynaecological origin by failure to demonstrate a purely transonic mass because of the gas contained within the bowel itself.

A haematoma of the rectus sheath may present as a very tender, painful swelling, wrongly diagnosed as a twisted ovarian cyst. In Glasgow a few of these cases have been correctly diagnosed, thus saving the patients from unnecessary operations.

It is usually possible to distinguish a fluid-filled ovarian cyst, from a urinary bladder with retention, because the lower border of the bladder appears to be 'open', being in shadow behind the symphysis pubis. In those cases where the bladder neck is displaced upwards by some tumour impacted within the pelvis, the pointed lower end indicates a trigone. This is totally uncharacteristic of any ovarian cyst.

Tumours within the bladder are very readily seen, especially sizeable papillomata and carcinomata. The latter usually demonstrate a fairly wide sessile base. In cases of postmenopausal bleeding in which the gynaecological findings are negative, sonar examination of the genito-urinary tract, including the bladder, is worthwhile as it may show an unsuspected origin for the blood loss.

Malignant parametrial infiltrations in patients with advanced carcinoma of the cervix may be evaluated by sonar. Using the full bladder technique, and first

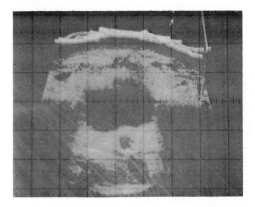 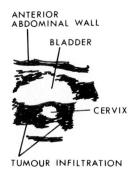

Fig. 4.21 Carcinoma of cervix, stage III. Transverse suprapubic view through full bladder shows cervix with infiltration on either side of it.

localizing the region of the internal os of the cervix, a careful transverse scan is made at the appropriate angle to visualize, as far as possible, parametrial infiltration, as shown in Fig. 4.21. This work is still in an early stage of development but promises to be of use, not only in staging a carcinoma of cervix, but in indicating response to radiotherapy.

4.12. FAILED IUCD AND EARLY PREGNANCY

It is not difficult to demonstrate the presence of an IUCD within the uterus [4.31]. What is particularly interesting is the study of these cases where the device has clearly failed to prevent pregnancy. In an impressive series [4.37] of 11 cases showing the coexistence of an IUCD and an intrauterine pregnancy, the device was always located below the gestation sac with a space in between, four of the devices in fact being so low in the lower uterine cavity as to suggest being in a state of partial expulsion. It would be interesting to know if the converse, namely of locating the IUCD properly situated in the upper uterine segment ensured greater protection for the wearer.

REFERENCES

4.1.   BARNETT, E. and MORLEY, P. (1971). Ultrasound in the investigation of space-occupying lesions of the urinary tract. *Br. J. Radiol.*, **44**, 733–42.

4.2.   BISHOP, E.H. (1966). Obstetric uses of the ultrasonic motion sensor. *Am. J. Obstet. Gynec.*, **96**, 863–7.

4.3.   CAMPBELL, S. (1968). An improved method of fetal cephalometry by ultrasound. *J. Obstet. Gynaec. Br. Commonw.*, **75**, 568–76.

4.4.   CAMPBELL, S. (1969). The prediction of fetal maturity by ultrasonic measurement of the biparietal diameter. *J. Obstet. Gynaec. Br. Commonw.*, **76**, 603–9.

4.5.   CAMPBELL, S. and DEWHURST, C.J. (1970). Quintuplet pregnancy diagnosed and assessed by ultrasonic compound scanning. *Lancet*, **1**, 101–3.

4.6.   CAMPBELL, S., PRYSE-DAVIES, J., COLTART, T.M., SELLAR, M.J. and SINGER, J.D. (1975). Ultrasonics in diagnosis of spina bifida. *Lancet*, **1**, 1065–72.

4.7.   CAMPBELL, S. and WILKIN, D. (1975). Ultrasonic measurement of fetal abdomen circumference in the estimation of fetal weight. *Br. J. Obstet. Gynaec.*, **82**, 689–97.

4.8.   COYLE, M.G., GREIG, M. and WALKER, J. (1962). Blood progesterone and urinary pregnanediol and oestrogens in foetal death from severe pre-eclampsia. *Lancet*, **2**, 275–7.

4.9.   DONALD, I. (1963). The use of ultrasonics in the diagnosis of abdominal swellings. *Br. med. J.*, **2**, 1154–5.

4.10. DONALD, I. (1965). Ultrasonic echo sounding in obstetrical and gynecological diagnosis. *Am. J. Obstet. Gynec.*, **93**, 935–41.

4.11. DONALD, I. (1965). Diagnostic uses of sonar in obstetrics and gynaecology. *J. Obstet. Gynaec. Br. Commonw.*, **72**, 907–19.

4.12. DONALD, I. (1968). Ultrasonics in obstetrics. *Br. med. Bull.*, **24**, 71–5.

4.13. DONALD, I. (1969). Sonar as a method of studying prenatal development. *J. Pediat.*, **75**, 326–33.

4.14. DONALD, I. (1971). Sonar. Further scope and prospects. *Proc. Roy. Soc. Med.*, **64**, 991–6.

4.15. DONALD, I. (1974). Limitations of present day sonar techniques in obstetrics and gynaecology. In *Ultrasonics in Medicine*, Ed. M. de Vlieger, D. N. White and V. R. McCready, pp. 7–13. Amsterdam: Excerpta Medica.

4.16. DONALD, I. (1974). New problems in sonar diagnosis in obstetrics and gynecology. *Am. J. Obstet. Gynec.*, **118**, 299–309.

4.17. DONALD, I. (1974). Apologia: how and why medical sonar developed. *Ann. Roy. Coll. Surg. Eng.*, **54**, 132–40.

4.18. DONALD, I. (1974). Sonar: what it can and cannot do in obstetrics. *Scot. med. J.*, **19**, 203–10.

4.19. DONALD, I. (1974). Sonar: the story of an experiment. *Ultrasound Med. Biol.*, **1**, 109–17.

4.20. DONALD, I. and ABDULLA, U. (1968). Placentography by sonar. *J. Obstet. Gynaec. Br. Commonw.,* **75**, 993–1006.

4.21. DONALD, I. and BROWN, T.G. (1961). Demonstration of tissue interfaces within the body by ultrasonic echo sounding. *Br. J. Radiol.,* **34**, 539–46.

4.22. DONALD, I., MACVICAR, J. and BROWN, T.G. (1958). Investigation of abdominal masses by pulsed ultrasound. *Lancet,* **1**, 1188–94.

4.23. DONALD, I., MORLEY P. and BARNETT, E. (1972). The diagnosis of blighted ovum by sonar. *J. Obstet. Gynaec. Br. Commonw.,* **79**, 304–10.

4.24. GOTTESFELD, K.R., THOMPSON, H.E., HOLMES, J. H. and TAYLOR, E.S. (1966). Ultrasonic placentography—a new method for placental localization. *Am. J. Obstet. Gynec.,* **96**, 538–47.

4.25. HANSMANN, M., VOIGT, U. and LANG, N. (1973). Ultraschall Messdaten als parameter zur Erkannung einer intrauterinen wachstumsretardierung. *Arch. Gynakologie,* **214**, 194–7.

4.26. HELLMAN, L.M., KOBAYASHI, M. and CROMB, E. (1973). Ultrasonic diagnosis of embryonic malformations. *Am. J. Obstet. Gynec.,* **115**, 615–23.

4.27. HIGGINBOTTOM, J., SALTER, J., PORTER, G. and WHITFIELD, C.R. (1975). Estimations of fetal weight from ultrasonic measurement of trunk circumference. *Br. J. Obstet. Gynaec.,* **82**, 698–701.

4.28. JOHNSON, W.L., STEGALL, H.F., LEIN, J.N. and RUSHMER, R.F. (1965). Detection of fetal life in early pregnancy with an ultrasonic Doppler flowmeter. *Obstet. Gynec., N.Y.,* **26**, 305–7.

4.29. KING, D.L. (1973). Placental migration demonstrated by ultrasonography. *Radiology,* **109**, 167–70.

4.30. MACVICAR, J. and DONALD, I. (1963). Sonar in the diagnosis of early pregnancy and its complications. *J. Obstet. Gynaec. Br. Commonw.,* **70**, 387–95.

4.31. PIIEROINEN, D. (1972). Ultrasonic localization of intrauterine contraceptive devices. *Acta obstet. gynec. scand.,* **51**, 203–7.

4.32. ROBINSON, H.P. (1972). Detection of fetal heart movement in first trimester of pregnancy using pulsed ultrasound. *Br. med. J.,* **4**, 466–8.

4.33. ROBINSON, H.P. (1973). Sonar measurement of fetal crown-rump length as a means of assessing maturity in the first trimester of pregnancy. *Br. med. J.,* **4**, 28–31.

4.34. ROBINSON, H.P. (1975). The diagnosis of early pregnancy failure by sonar. *Br. J. Obstet. Gynaec.,* **82**, 849–62.

4.35. ROBINSON, H.P. and FLEMING, J.E.E. (1975). A critical evaluation of sonar crown-rump length measurements. *Br. J. Obstet. Gynaec.,* **82**, 702–10.

4.36. SUNDÉN, B. (1964). On the diagnostic value of ultrasound in obstetrics and gynaecology. *Acta obstet. gynec. scand.,* **43**, suppl. 6.

4.37. TSAI, W.S., CHEN, W.Y., CHEN, Y.P. and WEI, P.Y. (1973). Sonographic visualization of co-existing gestation sac and I.U.C.D. in the uterus and a consideration of a causative factor of accidental pregnancy. *Internat. J. Fert.,* **18**, 85–92.

4.38. WILLOCKS, J., DONALD, I., DUGGAN, T.C. and DAY, N. (1964). Foetal cephalometry by ultrasound. *J. Obstet. Gynaec. Br. Commonw.,* **71**, 11–20.

4.39. WILLOCKS, J., DONALD, I., CAMPBELL, S. and DUNSMORE, I.R. (1967). Intrauterine growth assessed by ultrasonic foetal cephalometry. *J. Obstet. Gynaec. Br. Commonw.,* **74**, 639–47.

5. Ultrasonic investigations in ophthalmology

E.J. GIGLIO*

5.1. INTRODUCTION

The increased use of ultrasonic diagnosis in ophthalmology has led to its inclusion in the curriculum of ophthalmological residencies in the USA. Ultrasonic techniques augment information available by other methods, by elucidating the properties of lesions which are optically visible, and by adding and supplying data where direct observation is impossible. For example, in opaque cornea or cataract, or in orbital disease, ultrasound may provide information which cannot otherwise be obtained.

Ultrasound is also useful for axial measurement of tissue thickness, and for distance measurements within the eye. Thus, interest in the growth and development of the eye during childhood, and particularly in the process which tends to produce emmetropia, has required an independent method for the measurement of the axial dimensions of the eye, in order to supplement measurements by keratometry, purkinje, and slit lamp methods.

5.2. BIOMETRY

In addition to the principles described in Chapters 1 and 2, some special considerations are particularly relevant to ophthalmological investigations.

The validity of measurement along the anterior-posterior axis of the eye using ultrasound has been established [5.10, 5.12], and the method has been calibrated against test fixtures to show that it can be even more precise than optical or x-ray methods [5.8]. The stability of the measurements on humans over time is also detailed in the same report.

The use of ultrasound for measurement in the eye must consider the use to which the measurement will be put in order to determine the precision required. If the interest is in change of refraction of 0.25 D, as a result of posterior segment length change, then measurement to approximately 70 μm is required. In measurements of tissue thickness, it is desirable to detect changes of 1 per cent. One per cent of corneal thickness is about 5 μm, and those of retina or choroid are a little less than this.

If these values are accepted as reasonable measurement goals, then the use of ordinary diagnostic equipment is precluded by inadequate magnification and axial resolution. The normal 100 mm graticule of a CRT, using either single trace A-scan or B-scan can display the echoes from the eye with a magnification of

---

*Dr Giglio kindly contributed Sections 5.1 – 5.4. The remainder of this Chapter was written by the editor.

about 4×. Thus, an average eye of 25 mm length can occupy the full 100 mm of the screen, but this is insufficient for making measurements to 70 μm of axial length, or for evaluating changes in corneal thickness of 1 per cent. In addition it should be noted that A-scan instruments normally display the response of the transducer to the electrical pulse and this further reduces the length over which the eye echoes can be shown. Moreover, the early part of the time-base is unused (unless it is triggered after a delay) if a standoff is used in front of the transducer in order to see the front surface of the cornea.

In addition to the need for adequate magnification, interfaces such as retina, choroid, and sclera, which are separated by less than 0·5 mm require adequate axial resolution for their delineation. Frequencies of 6, 8, or even 10 MHz generally used for the display of space occupying lesions in the eye are usually not capable of resolving the complex of echoes from the rear of the eye. Higher frequencies with considerable damping are necessary, but increasing frequency and damping leads to rapid loss of penetration. The difficulty is helped, however, by the use of larger transducers with partial focusing. The problem of magnification and retaining maximum display space for the echoes from the eye can be solved in a number of ways. The transducer artifact and the space occupied by the standoff can be eliminated by gating, which causes the sweep of the oscilloscope to be triggered by the first reflexion from the eye, that is, by the front surface of the cornea. Since oscilloscopes are available with four channel 'plug in' amplifiers, the use of such an arrangement permits sequential triggering of each channel after an appropriate delay, and the display of all the interfaces from the eye with a magnification of about 20×. The sweep speed can then be 10 ns mm^{-1} and the thickness of the cornea, for example, occupies about 7 mm at the start of the trace.

It should be pointed out that good axial resolution requires that the pulse length should be as short as is consistent with the transfer of sufficient power to enable adequate reflexions to be returned from the rear of the eye. The equipment described here uses pulses of 65 ns with a repetition rate of 2000 s^{-1}.

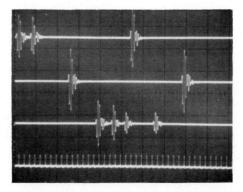

Fig. 5.1 Reflexions from nylon threads (38 μm diameter) stretched across the diameter of a hollow cylinder and spaced to mimic the interfaces in an eye. Top trace: front and rear of cornea and front of lens. Second trace: front and rear of lens. Third trace: front of retina, choroid, sclera, and rear of sclera. Fourth trace shows 0·25 μs time marks. Delays: at beginning of second trace, 3μs; at beginning of third trace, 30μs.

A number of instruments of this design have been built* and are in use. A more complete description has been reported previously [5.8]. Fig. 5.1 shows reflexions from a test block with 38 μm nylon threads, spaced approximately like the interfaces in the eye, used to validate the equipment.

Small movements of the eye may produce large changes in the received echoes. For example, it has been shown [5.2, 5.17] that translations of 0·5 mm produce significant changes in the displayed echoes. Even with fairly cooperative patients it is difficult for them to maintain sufficiently accurate fixation. The examination of the eye using A-scan has been described as a dynamically changing display. These facts further dictate the conditions required for making measurements in the eye. Aid must be supplied to provide more stable fixation. Several alternatives are available, including aids for the eye under test, aids for the companion eye, or a combination of both. A fibre optic may be placed in a hole drilled through the centre of the transducer along the axis of the ultrasonic beam, and the patient wears a goggle with normal saline between the transducer and the eye. In addition to the problem of leakage from the goggle, the eye is blurred by about 40 diopters due to loss of refracting power of the cornea. In spite of efforts to produce a very directional source, the recessed fibre optic in a carefully blackened hole behaves as though a secondary source were located at the edge of the opening and can be seen through a considerable angle (5°). The addition of fixation control for the companion eye is of help: if the eye not under test is directed to look through a tube (internal diameter about 5 mm, length 300 mm) placed 10—12 mm from the eye, fixation of a distant object controls accommodation and limits movement to less than 1°. The tube may be manipulated so that the light from the fibre optic is superimposed on the distant object (a cross) seen through the tube, and under these circumstances the blurred image of the fibre optic is very large compared to the hole containing the cross. With this arrangement the echoes from the eye are present on the oscilloscope face, but the transducer still has to be repositioned to obtain maximum amplitudes and maximum resolution. This is as should be expected: maximum amplitudes are to be obtained along the optic axis and not along the visual line, which may be several degrees from it.

If many measurements are to be made, the goggle method is not ideal. Other approaches used by investigators in this field include the following:

(i) Use of a cylindrical standoff with a contact lens flange supported by the sclera — patient supine [5.10]. Leakage, and possible distortion of the globe, are problems.

(ii) A cylindrical standoff sealed by a thin membrane [5.12]. Loss of position of front surface of cornea and variable thickness of coupling layer between membrane and cornea introduce error.

(iii) An alignment device in which the patient leans forward and places his eye into an eye cup [5.5]. The device aligns the transducer with the visual axis. No provision for adjustment is made to place the transducer along the optic axis.

*Automation Industries, Sperry Products Division, Shelter Rock Road, Danbury, Connecticut, USA.

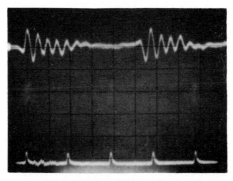

Fig. 5.2   Reflexions from the front and rear of cornea to demonstrate phase inversion. Thickness of cornea should be measured from first negative going indication of the first signal to the first positive going indication of the second signal. Changes of 1 per cent in corneal thickness are easily established. Lower trace shows 0·25 μs time marks.

(iv)   An automatic device to carry the transducer and standoff to the eye, coupling without touching and returning to its rest position in 72 ms [5.9]. Alignment with the visual axis is not difficult. Alignment with the optic axis is much more difficult.

(v)   A hand held probe designed for use with young children has had considerable success [5.7]. The device is conical, soft (silicone rubber), with a 4 mm opening, uncapped.

The problem of measurement involves the identification of the start of the disturbance reflected at the first interface, as well as the start of the disturbance reflected from the second interface, between which the time interval must be measured. Any cycle in the disturbance produced at the first interface could be used provided the same cycle in the second disturbance could be identified. For a number of reasons, the build-up time for the reflexion from the first interface need not be the same as that of the second. In addition, the half wavelength error which occurs if only positive or negative peaks are used must not be neglected: this phenomenon is due to the phase inversion which occurs when the characteristic impedance of the second medium is greater than that of the first. Fig. 5.2 shows reflexions from front and rear of the cornea. Measurement should be made from the negative going start of the first signal, to the positive going start of the second.

The measurement of the time interval has been accomplished in various ways, as follows:

(i) Visual reading from the oscilloscope with time-base graticule calibrated in time units.

(ii)   Superimposed scale which purports to convert time to distance.*

(iii)   A water interferometer, which seeks to equate a path length in water to the displayed time interval [5.10].

*The conversion from the measurement of time to the estimation of distance involves the assumption of velocity. The following values of velocity (in m s^{-1}) may be assumed, at 37°C: cornea, 1600; aqueous, 1532; lens, 1641; vitreous, 1532; retina, 1550; choroid, 1550; sclera, 1650.

(iv) Photograph of screen and measurement of photograph, assuming knowledge of overall magnification [5.12].

(v) Time marks generated on screen and photographed with the time interval: marks serve as time reference [5.8].

(vi) Counter with preset stop and start gates [5.5].

(vii) Timebase of oscilloscope replaced by variable frequency sinusoidal generator. When the period of generator is equal to the time interval to be measured, the signals representing the time interval to be measured overlap [5.16]. This method, with its opportunity for great magnification, permits the operator to judge when to start and to stop the measured interval; but it is better suited to a static than a dynamic situation.

(viii) A computing counter, interpolating the ambiguity produced by ± 1 count [5.11].

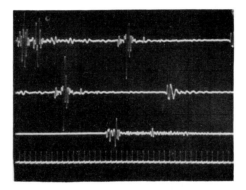

Fig. 5.3 Reflexions from a normal human eye obtained with use of uncapped conical standoff. Signals are not as 'clean' as those from threads but visual separations can be made even at the rear of the eye: this would be difficult with an electronic counter. Fourth trace shows $0.25 \mu s$ time marks. Delays: at beginning of second trace, $3 \mu s$; at beginning of third trace, $26 \mu s$.

The use of counters presents at least three difficulties. Firstly, in practical application the gates cannot be positioned to measure small intervals such as 0.5 mm for cornea or tissues at the rear of the eye—retina, choroid, and sclera. Secondly, special arrangement is required to trigger the counter with start and stop edges of opposite polarities, and the assumption of equal rise-times can contribute to error. Thirdly, the precisions of the start and stop can only be as good as the echo signals permit, and real echoes are not as '*clean*' as might be desired.

Fig. 5.3 is an example of reflexions obtained from a normal eye.

In summary, ultrasound as applied to measurement in the eye involves the use of appropriate equipment—pulser, receiver, transducer, display—and appropriate means for the application of the transducer, and adequate data reduction. It is natural to try to make these measurements as quickly and automatically as possible, but it is important to beware of errors. The expected error is often much less than the real error.

5.3. THE A-SCOPE IN INTRAOCULAR INVESTIGATIONS

Plane transducers of 3–8 mm in diameter, and frequencies of 6–12 MHz, are most often used. The probe is held in direct contact with the eye*, and either the tears, or a drop of a viscous solution of methylcellulose, provides the ultrasonic coupling. The examination of the eye using this method should be regarded as a *dynamic* examination, in which the decision of whether an abnormality is found, and, if so, what its nature may be, is made while the probe is in motion. A representative echogram showing the abnormality may later be photographed.

An A-scan of an eye affected by secondary detachment and tumour is shown in Fig. 5.4. The use of ultrasound for the detection of pathology in the eye requires that the examiner should be familiar with the anatomy, and with the normal pictures that are produced with his particular system. At the present time, it is not anticipated that the examination will be carried out by technicians. In skilled and experienced hands, a high degree of accuracy in diagnosis may be expected. The time required for an examination is usually about 5–15 min.

5.4. THE A-SCOPE IN ORBITAL INVESTIGATIONS

In the orbit, landmarks are fewer and less reliable than in the eye. Orbital fat undergoes compressions and deformations, and the optic nerve space changes position, as the eye changes its gaze. Nevertheless, some features can be distinguished ultrasonically. Bone attenuates ultrasound rapidly, and echoes are

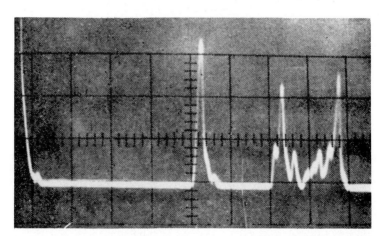

Fig. 5.4 A-scan showing secondary detachment and tumour. Made using 10 MHz system [5.13]. The lens was avoided in making this scan. The demodulated display shows (left to right) the echo from the sclera, the detached retina, and tumour echoes from a choroidal melanoma. The defect would be viewed from various angles to establish its certainty and its extent. The detached retina would be examined to determine its elevation, the organisation of the fluid behind it, and the possibility of a melanoma behind a flat detachment. A tumour of substantial thickness would be examined from two or more positions to substantiate that the large-amplitude echoes remain in the same relative positions with respect to the globe. A foreign body would be located in a like manner. (*Courtesy*: A. Oksala and *Am. J. Ophth.*)

*The eye is first anaesthetized with a drop of, for example, *Novesine* (0·4 per cent oxybuprocaine, 0·01 per cent chlorhexidine acetate).

not received from beyond the front surface of the orbital wall. Normal orbital tissues seem not to be differentiated. Only the globe, the optic nerve space, and the fatty orbital tissue, can be separately visualized.

Tumour tissue tends to attenuate ultrasound less rapidly than the normal tissue in the orbit. Consequently tumour echoes are relatively smaller, and the tumour can be circumscribed. In addition, a tumour is likely to be more stable and less compressible than normal tissues. Therefore, the globe may often be pushed in the direction of the suspected tumour, and the effect on the echogram can be observed. In a series [5.14] of 724 cases, satisfactory clinical proof of diagnosis was available in 357. Of those which were tumour-positive, the ultrasonic findings were 97 per cent correct; and of those which were tumour-negative, the ultrasonic predictions were 99 per cent correct. There are now established criteria by which tumours can be identified from their echograms [5.15].

5.5. TWO-DIMENSIONAL SCANNING IN OPHTHALMOLOGY

The first paper [5.1] describing ultrasonic two-dimensional visualization of the eye was published in 1958. A 15 MHz system was used, with the patient's eyes looking into the water bath, his face sealed by a rubber mask. The images produced by this instrument, and by some of those constructed later, reveal amazing detail of both the normal and abnormal anatomy of the eye and orbit. Whether such images are more helpful in patient care than the information which can be obtained with an A-scope by a skilled operator is open to question; but undoubtedly they are of enormous potential value because they are relatively easily interpreted.

Almost all two-dimensional ophthalmic scanners use water-bath coupling. The method is reliable and the results are clinically useful in the diagnosis of many kinds of ocular abnormalities [5.6]. Orbital scans are more difficult to interpret, but the ability to map out the position and extent of a tumour can be decisive in planning treatment.

Excellent results, some examples of which are shown in Fig. 5.5, have been obtained with a conventional abdominal contact scanner modified to visualize the eye through a water bath [5.18, 5.19, 5.20].

One exception to the usual water-bath type of scanner for ophthalmology has a hand-held housing with a thin plastic window, behind which a 7·5 MHz probe (focal length 15 mm) oscillates through an arc of approximately 30° [5.3]. The probe oscillation is provided by an electric motor driven at a sufficient speed to give an acceptable flicker-free display; the ultrasonic pulse repetition rate is 4000 s^{-1}. This real-time system gives good visualization of posterior globe and orbit [5.4].

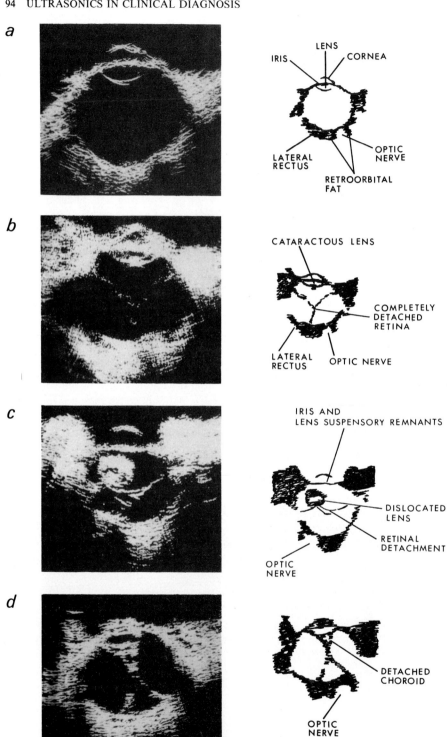

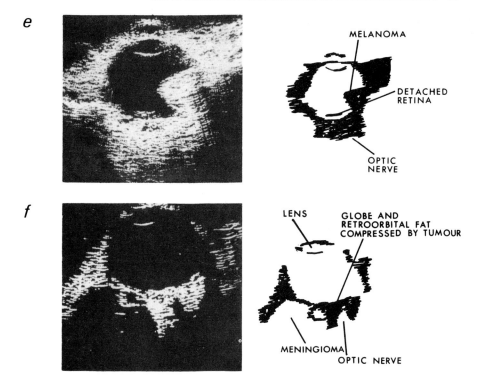

Fig. 5.5 Two-dimensional ultrasonic scans of the eye and orbit. (*a*) Normal.(*b*) Simple retinal detachment. (*c*) Traumatic retinal detachment with dislocated lens. (*d*) Complete choroidal detachment. (*e*) Choroidal melanoma. (*f*) Meningioma of lateral orbital wall. (*Courtesy*: G.R. Sutherland.)

Note: These scans were made with a Nuclear Enterprises Diasonograph type NE4102 (see Appendix). Water bath coupling was used: the frequency was 8 MHz.

REFERENCES

5.1. BAUM, G. and GREENWOOD, I. (1958). The application of ultrasonic locating techniques to ophthalmology. *Arch. ophthal.,* **60**, 263–79.

5.2. BAUM, G. and GREENWOOD, I. (1967). A critique of time amplitude ultrasonography. *Arch. ophthal.,* **65**, 367–71.

5.3. BRONSON, N.R. (1972). Development of a simple B-scan ultrasonoscope. *Trans. Am. ophthal. Soc.,* **70**, 365–408.

5.4. BRONSON, N.R. (1974). Contact B-scan ultrasonography. *Am. J. Ophthal.,* **77**, 181–91.

5.5. COLEMAN, D.J. and CARLIN, B. (1966). Transducer alignment and electronic measurement of visual axis dimensions in the human eye using time amplitude ultrasound. In *Ultrasonics in Ophthalmology,* Ed. A. Oksala and H. Gernet, pp. 204–14. Basel: Karger.

5.6. COLEMAN, D.J. and JACK, R.L. (1973). B-scan ultrasonography in diagnosis and management of retinal detachments. *Arch. ophthal.,* **90**, 29–34.

5.7. GIGLIO, E.J. and LUDLAM, W.M. (1971). A hand-held probe for acoustic coupling in ultrasonic intraocular distance measurements of young children. *Am. J. Optom.,* **48**, 1025–30.

5.8. GIGLIO, E.J., LUDLAM, W.M. and WITTENBERG, S. (1969). Improvement in the measurement of intraocular distances using ultrasound. *J. acoust. Soc. Am.,* **44**, 1359–64.

5.9. GIGLIO, E.J. and MEYERS, R.R. (1969). An automatic probe transport to the eye for ultrasound. *Am. J. Optom.,* **46,** 275–82.

5.10. JANSSON, F. (1963). Determination of the axis length of the eye roentgenologically and by ultrasound. *Acta ophthal.,* **41,** 236–46.

5.11. LACY, L.L. and DANIEL, A.C. (1972). Measurement of ultrasonic velocities using a digital averaging technique. *J. acoust. Soc. Am.,* **52,** 189–95.

5.12. LEARY, G., SORSBY, A., RICHARDS, M. and CHASTON, J. (1963). Ultrasonographic measurement of the components of ocular refraction in life—I. Technical considerations. *Vision Res.,* **3,** 487–95.

5.13. OKSALA, A. (1964). The clinical value of time-amplitude ultrasonography. *Am. J. Ophthal.,* **57,** 453–60.

5.14. OSSOINIG, K. (1969). Routine ultrasonography of the orbit. In *Ultrasonography in Ophthalmology,* Ed. M.A. Wainstock, pp. 613–42. Boston: Little, Brown.

5.15. OSSOINIG, K.C. (1974). Quantitative echography—an important aid for the acoustic differentiation of tissues. In *Ultrasonics in Medicine,* Ed. M. de Vlieger, D.N. White and V.R. McCready, pp. 49–54. Amsterdam: Excerpta Medica.

5.16. PAPADAKIS, E.P. (1967). Ultrasonic phase velocity by the pulse echo overlap method incorporating diffraction phase correction. *J. acoust. Soc. Am.,* **42,** 1045–51.

5.17. PURNELL, E. and SOKOLLU, A. (1962). An evaluation of time amplitude ultrasonography in ocular diagnosis. *Am. J. Ophthal.,* **54,** 1103–9.

5.18. SUTHERLAND, G.R. and FORRESTER, J.V. (1974). B-scan ultrasonography in ophthalmology. *Br. J. Radiol.,* **47,** 383–6.

5.19. SUTHERLAND, G.R. and FORRESTER, J.V. (1975). Demonstration of abnormalities of the lens by echography. *Br. J. Radiol.,* **48,** 1019–22.

5.20. SUTHERLAND, G.R., FORRESTER, J.V. and RAILTON, R. (1975). Echography in the diagnosis and management of retinal detachment. *Br. J. Radiol.,* **48,** 796–800.

FOR FURTHER READING

GIGLIO, E.J. and LUDLAM, W.M. (1966). Ultrasound—a diagnostic tool for examination of the eye. *Am. J. Optom.,* **43,** 687–731.

GITTER, K.A., KEENEY, A.H., SARIN, L.K. and MEYER, D. (Eds.) (1969). *Ophthalmic Ultrasound.* St. Louis: Mosby.

OKSALA, A. and GERNET, H. (Eds.) (1967). *Ultrasonics in Ophthalmology.* Basel: Karger.

VANYSÉK, J., PREISOVÁ, J. and OBRAZ, J. (1970). *Ultrasonography in Ophthalmology.* London: Butterworths.

WAINSTOCK, M.A. (Ed.) (1969). *Ultrasonography in Ophthalmology.* Boston: Little, Brown.

6. Ultrasonic investigation of the hepatobiliary system and the spleen

K.J.W. TAYLOR

6.1. LIVER

6.1.a. Introduction

Throughout the development of ultrasound techniques, there have been sporadic reports on the use of ultrasound in the diagnosis of liver disease [6.6., 6.14, 6.15, 6.16, 6.23, 6.24]. The technique has found application in the diagnosis of cirrhosis and especially in the differentiation of solid from cystic masses [6.26]. This has permitted successful diagnosis of cysts and abscesses of the liver [6.2, 6.41].

Ultrasound has been generally disappointing in the diagnosis of metastatic disease of the liver with the exception of isolated successful reports [6.15]. Thus, in 1970, a failure rate of 53 per cent in the detection of abnormality was reported [6.23] in patients with clinically obvious metastatic disease using conventional ultrasound equipment and it was concluded that isotope examination was a superior technique. The failure rate in a similar study [6.22] in 1973 was 39 per cent. Other workers have reported that ultrasound was of value in establishing normality in patients with equivocal liver isotope scan [6.10]. These difficulties result from limits imposed from the use of instrumentation basically designed for obstetric applications. For obstetric use, it is often sufficient to display the contour of the fetal head and the placental edge which are large discontinuities of characteristic impedance, and which therefore are the sites of large echoes. The modifications of the gray-scale technique, in which very low level echoes are displayed, has greatly increased the value of ultrasonic examination of the liver since the consistency of the organ is displayed in addition to the mere outline produced by conventional techniques [6.35].

Gray-scale ultrasonography was introduced in 1972 [6.19, 6.20], and has been most widely applied to obstetric examination in which fine intrafetal anatomy can be displayed [6.21]. The modifications include focused transducers, to enhance the lateral resolution, compression amplification signal processing, and suitable display systems. After addition of time gain control (TGC or swept gain), there is a range of some 60 dB in the amplitude of echoes to be displayed in the limited dynamic range of about 20 dB of the display system. In conventional ultrasound techniques, the low level echoes are suppressed and only the relatively large ones are displayed on a storage oscilloscope with a resultant black and white format showing little more than the contour of an organ. Gray-scale signal processing involves the selective amplification of the low level echoes which originate from interfaces within soft tissues, but because of the limited dynamic range of the display systems, the larger echoes must be increasingly compressed. Non-storage display units must be used if the quantitative data on echo amplitude are to be retained as a gray-scale format. A permanent record can best be obtained by exposing a film to a high-quality, non-storage oscilloscope, but the increasing use of scan converters on commercially available gray-scale systems is a practical alternative.

There is both theoretical and practical evidence that an important site of echo formation involves interfaces with collagen and other supporting tissue elements [6.7, 6.39]. Thus, for the practical purposes of interpreting gray-scale scans, the imaging of intrahepatic structure may be considered as the display of the fibrous skeleton of the organ. Space-occupying lesions are apparent as defects in this normal structure, while diffuse abnormalities are apparent in the pattern of the returned echoes. Most metastases are not detectable with the conventional technique because of the failure to display the normal consistency; therefore defects are not apparent. The gray-scale technique results in such enhanced resolution of small space-occupying lesions, that vascular pulsation begins seriously to degrade it. Therefore scanning techniques have been developed to overcome this limitation.

6.1.b.   Scanning techniques in gray-scale ultrasonography

Mainly specular echoes are displayed using conventional machines; the amplitudes of these echoes, by definition, are highly dependent on the angle of incidence. For this reason, compound scanning was introduced [6.5] in which the transducer is moved in a series of arcs around the abdominal surface, to ensure that the beam is at normal incidence in the plane of the scan to any reflecting

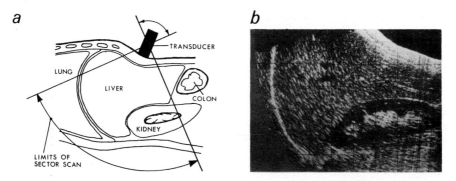

Fig. 6.1 (a) Diagram showing method of scanning liver using the 'acoustic window' between lung above and colon below. (b) Paramedian scan of liver and right kidney produced by the method illustrated in (a). Note that the consistency of the normal liver is displayed. (Courtesy: the Editors, *The British Journal of Radiology*.)

interface on at least one occasion during the scanning process. The beam may, however, be incident on a reflector on several occasions during the scan and this degrades resolution when the reflector is subject to vascular or respiratory excursions, since the reflector is registered in different positions of its oscillatory cycle. A further difficulty and potential source of error exists in the mechanical and electronic requirements for compounding, especially in the assumption that the velocity of ultrasound in different tissues is constant, which is necessary to register an interface with respect to the x and y axes.

One answer to the problem of organ movement is the use of real-time imaging techniques to enable reflectors to be imaged almost instantaneously. Unfortunately, in the present state of technical development of such systems, the resolution is not of the standard obtained by static imaging. Until improvements are made in the real-time imaging of abdominal organs, alternative techniques are simple sector and rectilinear scans [6.37]. In these techniques, the beam is only incident on each reflector on one occasion, so that any subsequent movement is irrelevant. The technique for liver examination is shown schematically in Fig. 6.1.a.

Although the amplitudes of specular echoes are highly dependent on angle of incidence, this is not true of the low-level echoes displayed by the gray-scale technique, which appear to be more omnidirectional [6.12]. This permits the non-compounded scanning techniques to be effective, but there is a further important sequel: the amplitudes of the echoes relate to the physical state of the tissue and are not merely dependent on the rather random orientation of the interface to the beam. This has great importance in the differential diagnosis of liver disease, and is also particularly apparent in the differential diagnosis of chronic splenomegaly [6.39]. This is considered later.

In clinical practice, a liver scan is carried out using the acoustic 'window' between the air-containing colon below, and the lung above (Fig. 6.1.a), so that the resultant scans (Fig. 6.1.b) are obtained in a series of parasagittal planes. The patient is requested to inspire deeply and the transducer is angled under the right costal margin using a suitable coupling agent such as mineral oil. The transducer is rotated smoothly through an arc and the scan can be continued into a simple linear scan of the abdomen if the liver, or any other mass, extends below the costal margin. This technique permits more of the right lobe of the liver to be displayed than the alternative intercostal and subcostal techniques described by other authors [6.6, 6.14]. Occasionally, the lateral parts of the liver are inaccessible due to air in the transverse colon and repeated attempts following mild purgation are worthwhile. The structures visualized by the technique include the liver, right hemidiaphragm, and right kidney, as shown in Fig. 6.1.b.

6.1.c. Visualization of liver by gray-scale ultrasonography

(i) *The normal liver*
The scans shown here were produced on a custom-built machine constructed on principles outlined elsewhere [6.17]. Equipment of similar quality, however, is becoming commercially available. The frequency is 3 MHz, with a swept gain rate of $2 \cdot 5$ dB cm^{-1}. For large individuals, or for patients with cirrhosis, a 2 MHz transducer may be used to advantage. The appearances of the normal liver depend on the plane of the parasagittal section and considerable experience is required to define the limits of normality.

A parasagittal section taken 20 mm to the left of the midline is seen in Fig. 6.2, showing the aorta posteriorly and the left lobe of the liver anteriorly. Note the normal structure through the entire liver substance. A parasagittal section 20 mm to the right of the midline (Fig. 6.3) shows the lumen of the inferior vena cava in longitudinal section. Again, the normal liver substance can be seen and the

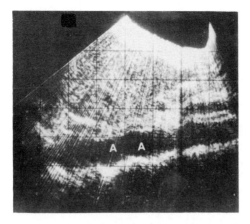

Fig. 6.2 Paramedian scan 10 mm to the left of the midline showing normal liver consistency with aorta (A) posteriorly.

portal vein appears as a straight vessel ascending to the hilum of the liver. Portal hypertension is associated with abnormalities in the size and form of the portal vein, that permit a non-intrusive diagnosis to be made.

(ii) *Discrete liver abnormalities*

Cystic lesions. Ultrasound is particularly successful in the differentiation of solid from cystic space-occupying lesions [6.26]. Polycystic disease can easily be diagnosed [6.6, 6.17], but smaller cystic lesions can also be displayed, as shown in Fig. 6.4. The characteristic appearances of a benign cyst include regular walls, an absence of echoes within the lesion, and overcompensation for depth attenuation distal to the lesion. The amplitudes of echoes within cysts are often best judged from the appearance of the A-scan. Since there is virtually no attenuation through the contents of a cyst, the addition of the standard swept gain results in

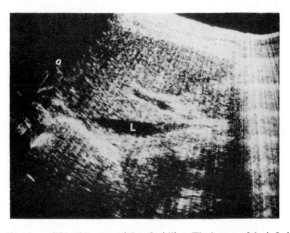

Fig. 6.3 Paramedian scan of liver 20 mm to right of midline. The lumen of the inferior vena cava (L) is seen posterior to the liver and the portal vein ascends to the porta hepatis.

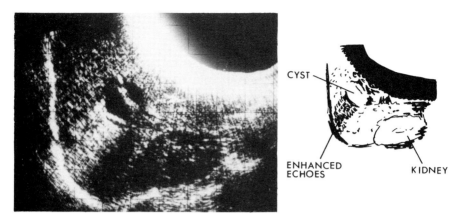

Fig. 6.4 Paramedian scan 50 mm to right of midline showing a 30 mm diameter benign cyst in the liver substance. Note the increased echoes posterior to the lesion confirming the fluid content. The displayed anatomy is comparable to that seen in Fig. 6.1.b.

overamplification of the echoes beyond the cyst and this is apparent on the resultant B-scan. In obese patients, some echoes may be seen in the cavity, perhaps due to 'tissue reverberations', and comparison with the echoes produced by the bladder content can be a useful internal calibration. For comparative purposes, two types of malignant cysts are considered later.

Abscesses. Ultrasound is a valuable modality for the diagnosis of subphrenic and intrahepatic abscesses. It is fortunate that left subphrenic abscesses can be easily diagnosed by radiological methods while right subphrenics are easily displayed by ultrasound. The characteristic ultrasound finding is an area returning abnormally low level echoes, the amplitude depending on the fluidity of the abscess contents. There is usually evidence of overcompensation for depth attenuation, but there may be considerable difficulty in distinguishing between

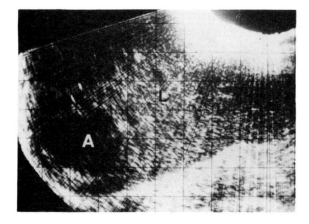

Fig. 6.5 Paramedian scan of liver (L) showing diffuse abnormality of the liver consistency with coarse, high level echoes, consistent with cholangitis. An abscess cavity (A) is seen high under the right hemidiaphragm.

partially necrotic tumours and abscesses. Surrounding evidence of coarse, high level echoes throughout the liver substance, strongly support the diagnosis of an inflammatory process. A small intrahepatic abscess situated high in the right lobe of the liver is seen in Fig. 6.5, and was found when the patient failed to improve after an emergency cholecystectomy for an empyema of the gallbladder. The coarse, high level echoes throughout the liver substance are consistent with ascending cholangitis and subsequent formation of the displayed abscess. The appearances of hydatid cysts seem to be specific (Fig. 6.6). Abscess cavities of daughter cysts are seen which return very low level echoes, almost simulating polycystic disease, but there are also areas of high level echoes, indicating an inflammatory process. Hydatid abscess cavities have been seen which extend through the diaphragm into the pleural space in patients who are remarkably well clinically.

Discrete malignant lesions. Over 4000 patients with suspected metastatic involvement of the liver had been scanned at The Royal Marsden Hospital up to the summer of 1975. The results show that, in experienced hands, the technique can be highly accurate and yield more informative data than that obtained by alternative techniques. The commonest sign of a liver metastasis consists of an area returning echoes of slightly lower amplitude than the normal tissue. The abnormality is most easily detected by turning down the intensity control on the storage oscilloscope monitor until the normal tissue is just registered, and the abnormal areas of malignant replacement are not registered at all. On the gray-scale display, the abnormal areas may be only a slightly darker shade of gray and less apparent. More diffuse malignancy is seen due to heterogeneity in the amplitude of the returned echoes, often associated with hepatomegaly.

Some types of tumours produce highly characteristic appearances in the liver. Hodgkins' disease and the lymphomas are highly homogeneous tumours producing very low level echoes that may simulate an abscess cavity, as shown in Fig.

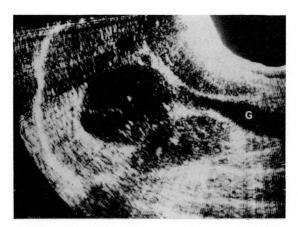

Fig. 6.6 Paramedian scan of liver showing cystic lesion with surrounding irregular high level echoes. The appearances are those of hydatid disease with daughter cysts. The gallbladder lumen (G) is seen anterior to the right kidney. (Courtesy: the Editors, *The British Journal of Radiology.*)

6.7.a. They have low attenuation so that some overcompensation for depth attenuation may be seen. Similar appearances are often found in metastases from coli-rectal primaries and 'oat cell' carcinoma of the bronchus. Due to the large difference in echo amplitude between these tumours and normal tissue, such metastases are most easily detected.

The ability to display small tumours in the liver substance by a non-intrusive technique enables chemotherapy to be instituted at an earlier stage in the dissemination process. Repeated examinations permit the response to treatment to be monitored. The liver with lymphomatous infiltration (Fig. 6.7.a) was re-

a   b

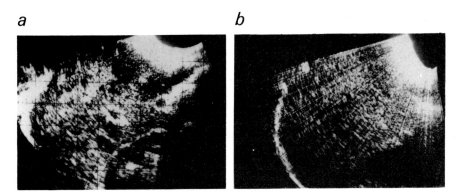

Fig. 6.7 (*a*) Paramedian scan of liver (compare Fig. 6.1.b) showing normal areas interspersed by multiple defects of more homogeneous tumour material. These appearances are consistent with infiltration by lymphoma or Hodgkins' disease. (*b*) Paramedian scan of liver of same patient after two months' chemotherapy and a marked improvement in the clinical state. Note that the consistency appears more normal.

scanned after two months of successful chemotherapy (Fig. 6.7.b). A less abnormal liver consistency is immediately apparent and this correlates well with the clinical improvement. Successful treatment of liver metastases may result in areas returning high level echoes which are consistent with fibrous replacement of tumour material. Thus, the ultrasound scan can be used to monitor the response of metastases to chemotherapy [6.8].

Malignant cysts may be found in the liver substance and have been seen most frequently in patients with carcinoma of the breast. They are characterized by irregular walls and return low level echoes due to contained cellular debris [6.16, 6.30]. The differentiation between benign and malignant cysts may present considerable difficulty in the obese in whom serial examination may be of great value. Necrotic, cystic tumours appear rather different from the secreting metastatic cystadendocarcinoma. These tumours appear as cystic masses on the surface of the liver showing local invasion, as shown in Fig. 6.8.a. Low level echoes are frequently returned due to debris in the pseudomucinous, or serous, contents. Thus, the appearances are those of a superficial, malignant liver cyst, almost invariably of ovarian origin. Immediate examination of the pelvis in these patients reveals the primary tumour (Fig. 6.8.b), lying posterior to the bladder. From consideration of the pathology, it seems almost certain that these tumours are peritoneal deposits invading the liver after transcoelomic spread.

a   *b*

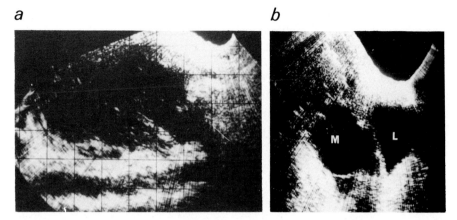

Fig. 6.8 (*a*) Paramedian scan 10 mm to left of midline (compare Fig. 6.2) showing liver substance
invaded and replaced by large, superficial cyst. The appearances are consistent with
metastatic cystadenocarcinoma. (*b*) Sagittal pelvic scan of same patient. The bladder lumen
(L) is seen with a cystic mass (M) above and behind it. These appearances are consistent with
a serous cystadenocarcinoma, almost certainly of the ovary. (Courtesy: the Editors, *The
British Journal of Radiology*.)

(iii) *Diffuse liver disease*

It is particularly in the differential diagnosis of diffuse liver disease that gray-
scale ultrasonography has much to offer as a non-invasive technique. Cirrhosis
has been reliably diagnosed by conventional ultrasound [6.15, 6.16] and it has
been shown that the cirrhotic liver returns higher level echoes than the normal
organ [6.25]. These early results on the value of ultrasound in diffuse liver disease
have been extended as a result of the enhanced resolution resulting from the use
of the gray-scale technique [6.38].

The appearances of cirrhosis vary with the degree of the pathology. In severe
cirrhosis, attenuation may be so high that the deeper parts of the liver are only

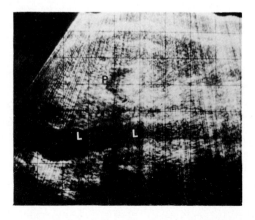

Fig. 6.9 Paramedian liver scan (compare Fig. 6.3) showing tortuous portal vein (P) in a patient with
known portal hypertension due to cirrhosis. The liver produces scattered, high level echoes
consistent with the diagnosis. The lumen of the inferior vena cava (L) is seen posteriorly.

reached by examination at a lower frequency (1—2 MHz). The appearances are those of very high level echoes distributed in a scattered pattern, as shown in Fig. 6.9. The portal vein is usually apparent and may be abnormally large. The shape of the portal vein is important, for, in proven cases of portal hypertension, the portal vein seems to be tortuous, often forming a comma-shaped vessel at the hilum of the liver [6.34]. Its characteristic shape enables it to be distinguished from an enlarged common bile duct. If portal hypertension is suspected, the spleen should be examined along the tenth interspace. Splenomegaly, consequent to portal hypertension, is immediately apparent.

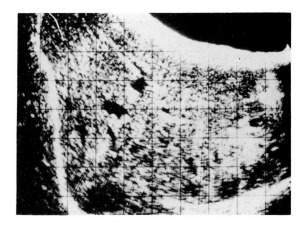

Fig. 6.10 Paramedian liver scan (compare Fig. 6.1.b) showing enlargement of the liver and well defined, very high level echoes. The vessels are unusually prominent. The appearances are those of fatty infiltration and chronic venous congestion.

Fatty infiltration without any marked fibrotic changes, also produces high level echoes but these are distributed in a more uniform pattern, as shown in Fig. 6.10. The liver is enlarged, and dilated vessels are apparent. Such appearances are usually described at subsequent post-mortem as venous congestion with fatty infiltration. They are seen fairly frequently in patients with carcinoma of the bronchus, who have been referred for investigation of the liver because of hepatomegaly. Therefore it is important that these benign changes are distinguished from malignant involvement.

Various other patterns of high level echoes are seen in different liver pathologies. Viral hepatitis and drug-induced jaundice are accompanied by increased peri-portal echoes and a biliary system of normal calibre [6.36]. The coarse high echoes seen in cholangitis, as illustrated in Fig. 6.4, have already been noted. A further benign change has been seen in some patients with lymphomas who, in biopsy, are found to have peri-portal lymphocytic infiltration. The patient whose scan is shown in Fig. 6.11.a was also jaundiced, and it is interesting to note that

a   b

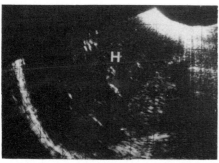 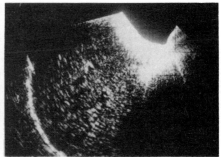

Fig. 6.11 (a) Paramedian liver scan (compare Fig. 6.1.b) showing intensely homogeneous liver (H)
found in benign, cellular infiltration of the liver. The liver is slightly enlarged.
(b) Paramedian liver scan of same patient after two months' chemotherapy. The liver size
has diminished and a 'normal' consistency is apparent. (Courtesy: the Editor, *Clinical
Radiology* and Glees *et al* [6.9].)

the jaundice resolved after two courses of chemotherapy while the liver ultrasound showed a decrease in the size of the liver and an increase in echo amplitude
to normal after this treatment. This is shown in Fig. 6.11.b. On first examination,
it might be considered that the intense homogeneity of the liver substance seen in
this scan was consistent with malignant replacement. A useful point in this
differentiation, however, is the uniformity of the changes in the benign pathology, whereas the malignant state tends to be more heterogeneous in appearance.

(iv) *Accuracy in the diagnosis of liver disease*
The accuracy varies markedly with the experience of the operator and with the
type of patient. If, for example, patients are selected for follow-up on the basis of
a post-mortem examination soon after the scan, fairly advanced pathology will
be present.

One hundred and twenty patients were followed after ultrasound and isotope
examinations [6.32]; diagnostic data were obtained in 82 per cent, while
contributory data were supplied in a further 10 per cent. These results were far
superior to Tc^{99m} sulphur colloid liver scans which can seldom contribute to the
differential diagnosis of space-occupying lesions.

Ultrasound findings have been compared with those of isotope examination
and needle and wedge biopsies of the liver in 52 patients with Hodgkins' disease
and non-Hodgkins' lymphomas [6.9]. It was found that ultrasound was especially valuable in excluding liver involvement for which an accuracy of 78 per
cent was attained. The remaining 22 per cent were false negatives. This compares
with 61 per cent false negatives by isotope examination. This was a group of
patients in whom any apparent liver disease would have excluded them from
laparotomy so that the liver pathology tended to be minimal and was only
present in 12 per cent of those undergoing laparotomy. Thus, the ultrasound
prediction of liver involvement of 56 per cent, which appears unremarkable,
must be compared with an accuracy of only 33 per cent for multiple needle
biopsies.

In another study [6.28], 70 patients with recurrent disease were followed after presentation with carcinoma of the breast. The liver ultrasound examination was compared with the prediction of involvement based on clinical examination, alkaline phosphatase estimation, and isotope examination. Ultrasound was superior to all other techniques for excluding liver involvement, and was also superior to clinical examination and isotope studies in predicting involvement.

Although these results are based on full time experience in ultrasound techniques, further improvements can be expected, both from increased experience and from technical modifications. It is already apparent, however, that the gray-scale technique promises to be a useful tool in the investigation of liver disease.

(v) *Liver biopsy*

The ability to display the liver consistency in increasing detail permits closed liver biopsy, an otherwise notoriously inaccurate procedure, to be performed on any area with an abnormal ultrasound pattern. This has been achieved with considerable success by the group in Copenhagen [6.27]. Since the liver moves considerably with vascular pulsation, however, a real-time, continuous imaging display for this procedure would make the technique considerably easier. As technical modifications become available, the applications for them, such as ultrasonically-guided liver biopsy, should greatly increase.

(vi) *Liver volume estimation*

The liver volume can be estimated from the areas of a series of longitudinal sections through the liver which can be integrated into a volume [6.18]. The irregular shape of the liver implies that the calculations are not simple and are best made on a computer. A simple, and clinically valuable alternative, is to measure the distance from the upper to the lower borders of the liver in a given plane, producing a measurement which may be compared on serial scans over a period of time.

6.2. BILIARY SYSTEM

A major reason for imaging the biliary system is to differentiate between intra- and extrahepatic causes for cholestatic jaundice, and this may present a difficult diagnostic problem. Current radiological methods include oral and intravenous cholangiography, but these are unlikely to be successful if the serum bilirubin exceeds 3 mg per cent [6.29]. Percutaneous cholangiography carries a significant risk of biliary peritonitis and therefore is usually only carried out immediately preoperatively. The new technique of endoscopic retrograde cholangiopancreatography (ERPC) is successful and diagnostic in 90 per cent of jaundiced patients [6.4] but it is intrusive and requires considerable manual dexterity. Laparotomy and liver biopsy are highly diagnostic but may precipitate liver failure if performed soon after the onset of jaundice [6.3, 6.11]. In this situation, a non-intrusive technique is a valuable addition, and ultrasound appears to be highly accurate.

Early workers considered that intrahepatic causes of jaundice could be differentiated from extrahepatic causes, but their subsequent experience did not

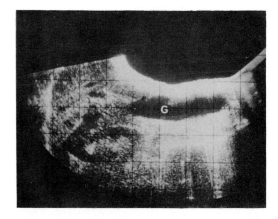

Fig. 6.12 Paramedian liver scan. A grossly dilated gallbladder (G) is seen while dilated biliary vessels are apparent in the liver substance.

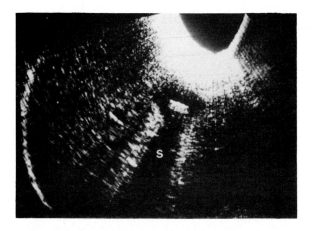

Fig. 6.13 Paramedian liver scan showing single gallstone in the gallbladder, which throws a marked shadow (S) posterior to it due to high attenuation by the stone.

confirm this [6.23, 6.24]. Dilated gallbladders and gallstones have been noted, and these observations may frequently be helpful in the diagnosis of extrahepatic jaundice. The gallbladder may not communicate with the remainder of the biliary tree, however, so that conclusions based on its dimension may be spurious, and it is the state of the biliary canaliculi, hepatic ducts and the common bile duct which is most valuable. These vessels have been imaged using the real-time technique [6.42] and, with enhanced resolution, by the gray-scale technique [6.33, 6.34, 6.36].

6.3.   GALLBLADDER

The dilated gallbladder is essentially a superficial cyst, and therefore is easily displayed on almost any B-scan machine. A grossly dilated gallbladder, due to chronic pancreatitis, is seen in Fig. 6.12. The biliary vessels are abnormally dilated, which implies that the gallbladder is not merely a mucocoele but that there is more proximal biliary obstruction.

Gallstones are well visualized, as shown in Fig. 6.13, even when they are not radio-opaque, and an important diagnostic feature is the marked shadowing effect beyond the stone, due to high attenuation of the beam by the stone. This shadow may be more obvious than the stone, but care must be exercised since the spiral valve arrangement at the neck of the gallbladder throws a shadow in all normal patients, which must not be confused with that due to a stone [6.34]. Care must also be taken to exclude shadowing from air in the transverse colon. No figures are available for the accuracy with which gallstones can be detected, but since this is a tomographic technique, small stones are easily missed.

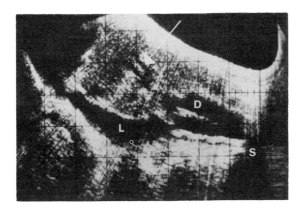

Fig. 6.14 Paramedian liver scan (compare Fig. 6.3) showing lumen of inferior vena cava posteriorly (L). The dilated common bile duct (D) has a characteristic shape and appearance and can be traced to the region of the duodenum below. There is dilatation of the intrahepatic biliary vessels (arrowed) which are diagnostic of extrahepatic biliary obstruction even if the common bile duct cannot be visualized. Biliary obstruction was due to carcinoma of the ampulla of Vater in which a gallstone was impacted. The presence of the gallstone may be inferred from the shadow (S).

A dilated common bile duct may be well seen in some patients (Fig. 6.14) on a paramedian section taken 20 mm to the right of the midline. If this can be traced inferiorly, the exact site of the extrahepatic biliary obstruction may be seen. In Fig. 6.14, the dilated common bile duct can be traced for 70 mm below the porta hepatis, which is the entire length of the duct. There is a shadow at the lower end of the duct due to a stone impacted in the ampulla of Vater. Although this permitted correct differentiation between extra- and intrahepatic causes of cholestatic jaundice, this report was not diagnostic since the stone was impacted at that site due to a carcinoma of the ampulla. On such sections, 25 cases of carcinoma of the pancreas have been successfully found. In patients who have been bedridden before referral, however, air in the transverse colon often prevents adequate visualization of the pancreatic region. Purgation is justified by the potential value of the diagnostic data, compared with the intrusion involved with alternative techniques. It is virtually always possible to display the liver substance near the midline, and the H-shaped configuration of the dilated biliary vessels (arrowed in Fig. 6.14) is diagnostic of biliary dilatation. These small vessels are not displayed if they are of normal calibre. This observation has permitted a correct diagnosis to be made in 64 out of 66 patients coming to laparotomy with extrahepatic biliary obstruction. Equally important, an intrahepatic cause of cholestatic jaundice was correctly predicted in a further 38 patients [6.40]. Technical limitations may make a definitive diagnosis difficult or impossible, but this basic differentiation between obstruction at the level of the small biliary vessels, or of the large ones, should become one of the more important applications for diagnostic ultrasound.

6.4. SPLEEN

The volume of the spleen has been estimated from serial transverse scans made at 20 mm intervals, and a good correlation with spleen weight has been attained

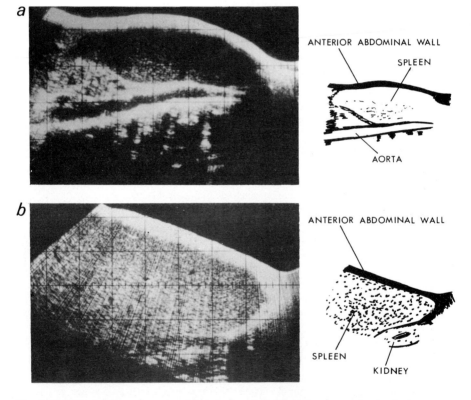

Fig. 6.15 (a) Paramedian spleen scan with aorta posteriorly. The spleen returns low level echoes deeply due to standard swept gain, but is relatively homogeneous. The appearances are those of treated leukaemia. In the absence of treatment, the low level echoes are not recorded. The appearances vary with the swept gain rate, which, therefore, is kept constant. (b) Paramedian spleen scan showing left kidney posteriorly. Note evenly distributed, very high level echoes throughout the spleen substance, with constant swept gain rate. These appearances nearly always indicate a non-malignant, chronic inflammatory cause of splenomegaly. This patient was found to have brucellosis.

[6.18]. It has been noted from the use of conventional machines, that no specific patterns have been described in association with any particular pathology [6.1]. The spleen returns very low level echoes, however, so that gray-scale techniques are essential for examination of the splenic consistency since these are the only contemporary machines in which the low level data are retained and displayed. Even then, better signal-to-noise ratio is required for the reliable differentiation of malignant involvement of the spleen.

Three categories of splenic consistency have been described [6.39]. Marked splenomegaly, which returns very low level echoes, and hence appears large and black, as shown in Fig. 6.15.a, has only been seen to date in malignant causes of splenomegaly, namely lymphomas and leukaemias. There is a group of diseases causing splenomegaly in which medium level echoes are seen. This group consists of benign diseases, and includes splenomegaly due to portal hypertension, myelofibrosis, and non-tropical splenomegaly. A third group includes inflammatory causes of splenomegaly such as tuberculosis, brucellosis, sarcoidosis and malaria. These return very high level echoes so that the splenic consistency appears white, as shown in Fig. 6.15.b. Myeloproliferative disorders, in which considerable amounts of collagen may be present, simulate a chronic inflammatory state and, occasionally, lymphomas may also do so.

These three groups of splenic consistencies are only the earliest observations, but do indicate that the gray-scale technique shows some promise in the differential diagnosis of chronic splenomegaly; this is a difficult diagnostic problem with alternative methods. It is also obvious that, in the development of a chronic inflammatory state, the splenic consistency shows a progressive change. This stresses the need for a quantitative technique so that progressive pathology in liver or spleen can be measured by serial scans. This could be of particular value in monitoring the effect of industrial exposure to hepato-toxic agents.

Various analytical techniques are under investigation to extract more quantitative data from the interrogation of tissues by an ultrasound beam and, in view of the quantity of data available, computer techniques may be required for data reduction. The amplitude of the A-scan can be analysed and this has been found to be significantly increased in cirrhosis [6.25]. In a similar way, the three categories of splenic consistency can be separately differentiated [6.39]. In the diagnosis of liver disease, however, the spatial distribution of the echoes may have equal importance to their amplitude.

In the present state of knowledge, ultrasonic examination of liver and spleen is still an art; but the increasing use of quantitative techniques should lead to more precise diagnosis and less dependence on operator experience and bias.

REFERENCES

6.1. BARNETT, E. and MORLEY, P. (1974). The spleen. In *Abdominal Echography,* p. 31. London: Butterworths.

6.2. BUTLER, T.J. and MCCARTHY, C.F. (1969). Pyogenic liver abscess. *Gut,* **10,** 389–99.

6.3. BOURKE, J.B., CANNON, P. and RITCHIE, H.D. (1967). Laparotomy for jaundice. *Lancet,* **2,** 521.

6.4. COTTON, P.B. (1972). Cannulation of the papilla of Vater by endoscopy and retrograde cholangiopancreatography (ERCP). *Gut,* **13,** 1014–25.

6.5. DONALD, I., MACVICAR, J. and BROWN, T.G. (1958). Investigation of abdominal masses by pulsed ultrasound. *Lancet*, **1**, 1188–94.
6.6. EVANS, K.T., MCCARTHY, C.F., READ, A.E.A. and WELLS, P.N.T. (1966). Ultrasound in the diagnosis of liver disease. *Br. med. J.*, **2**, 1368–9.
6.7. FIELDS, S. and DUNN, F. (1973). Correlation of echographic visualizability of tissue with biological composition and physiological state. *J. acoust. Soc. Am.*, **54**, 809–12.
6.8. GILBY, E.D. and TAYLOR, K.J.W. (1975). Ultrasound monitoring of hepatic metastases during chemotherapy. *Br. med. J.*, **1**, 371–3.
6.9. GLEES, J.P., TAYLOR, K.J.W., GAZET, J.C., PECKHAM, M.J. and MCCREADY, V.R. (1976). Accuracy of gray-scale ultrasonography of liver and spleen in Hodgkins' disease and the other lymphomas compared with isotope scans. *Clin. Radiol.*, in press.
6.10. GROS, C., WALTER, J.P. and PARISOT, B. (1972). Echography in liver pathology. *J. Radiol. Electrol. Med. Nucl.*, **53**, 740–1.
6.11. HARVILLE, D.D. and SUMMERSKILL, W.H.J. (1963). Surgery in acute hepatitis; causes and effects. *J. Am. med. Ass.*, **257**, 184.
6.12. HILL, C.R. (1974). Interactions of ultrasound with tissues. In *Ultrasound in Medicine*, ed. M. de Vlieger, D.N. White and V.R. McCready, pp. 14–20. Amsterdam: Excerpta Medica.
6.13. HILL, C.R. and CARPENTER, D.A. (1976). Ultrasonic echo imaging of tissue: instrumentation. *Br. J. Radiol.*, **49**, 238–43.
6.14. HOLM, H.H. (1971). Ultrasonic scanning in the diagnosis of space-occupying lesions of the upper abdomen. *Br. J. Radiol.*, **44**, 24–36.
6.15. HOLMES, J.H. (1966). Ultrasonic diagnosis of liver disease. In *Diagnostic Ultrasound*, ed. C.C. Grossman, J.H. Holmes, C. Joyner and E.W. Purnell, pp. 249–65. New York: Plenum Press.
6.16. HOWRY, D.H. (1965). A brief atlas of diagnostic ultrasonic radiologic results. *Radiol. Clin. N. Am.*, **3**, 433–52.
6.17. IGAWA, K. and MIYAGISHI, T. (1972). The use of scintillation and ultrasonic-scanning to disclose polycystic kidneys and liver. *J. Urol.*, **108**, 685–8.
6.18. KARDEL, T., HOLM, H.H., RASMUSSEN, S.N. and MORTENSEN, T. (1971). Ultrasonic determination of liver and spleen volume. *Scand. J. clin. lab. Invest.*, **27**, 123–8.
6.19. KOSSOFF, G. (1972). Improved techniques in ultrasonic cross-sectional echography. *Ultrasonics*, **10**, 221–7.
6.20. KOSSOFF, G. (1974). Display techniques in ultrasound pulse echo investigations: a review. *J. clin. Ultrasound*, **2**, 61–72.
6.21. KOSSOFF, G. and GARRETT, W.J. (1972). Ultrasonic film echography in gynecology and obstetrics. *Obstet. Gynec., N.Y.*, **40**, 229–305.
6.22. LEYTON, B., HALPERN, S., LEOPOLD, G. and HAGEN, S. (1973). Correlation of ultrasound and colloid scintiscan studies of the normal and disease liver. *J. nucl. Med.*, **14**, 27–33.
6.23. MCCARTHY, C.F., DAVIES, E.R., WELLS, P.N.T., ROSS, F.G.M., FOLLETT, D.H., MUIR, K.M. and READ, A.E. (1970). Comparison of ultrasonic and isotopic scanning in the diagnosis of liver disease. *Br. J. Radiol.*, **43**, 100–9.
6.24. MCCARTHY, C.F., READ, A.E.A., ROSS, F.G.M. and WELLS, P.N.T. (1967). Ultrasonic scanning of the liver. *Quart. J. Med.*, **36**, 517–24.
6.25. MOUNTFORD, R.A. and WELLS, P.N.T. (1972). Ultrasonic liver scanning: the A-scan in the normal and in cirrhosis. *Phys. Med. Biol.*, **17**, 261–9.
6.26. OSTRUM, B.J., GOLDBERG, B.B. and ISARD H.J. (1967). A-mode ultrasound differentiation of soft tissue masses. *Radiology*, **88**, 745–9.
6.27. RASMUSSEN, S.N., HOLM, H.H. KRISTENSEN, J.K. and BARLEBO, H. (1972). Ultrasonically guided liver biopsy. *Br. med. J.*, **2**, 500–2.
6.28. SMITH, I.A., TAYLOR, K.J.W., PECKHAM, M.J., GAZET, J.C., and MCCREADY, V.R., (1976). Comparison of gray-scale ultrasound with other methods for detection of liver metastases from carcinoma of the breast. *J. clin. Oncol.*, in press.
6.29. SUTTON, D. (Ed.). (1969). *Textbook of Radiology*, p. 711. Edinburgh: Livingstone.
6.30. TAYLOR, K.J.W. (1974). Ultrasonic patterns of tumors of the liver. *J. clin. Ultrasound*, **2**, 74–6.
6.31. TAYLOR, K.J.W. (1975). Gray-scale ultrasound imaging: diagnosis of metastatic cystadeno-carcinoma of ovary. *Br. J. Radiol.*, **48**, 937–9.
6.32. TAYLOR, K.J.W. and CARPENTER, D.A. (1974). Comparison of radioisotope and ultrasound examination in the investigation of hepatobiliary disease. In *Ultrasound in Medicine*, ed. D. White, vol. 1, pp. 159–67. New York: Plenum Press.
6.33. TAYLOR, K.J.W. and CARPENTER, D.A. (1974). Gray-scale ultrasonography in the investigation of obstructive jaundice. *Lancet*, **2**, 586–7.

6.34. TAYLOR, K.J.W. and CARPENTER, D.A. (1975). The anatomy and pathology of the porta hepatis and biliary tree demonstrated by gray-scale ultrasonography. *J. clin. Ultrasound,* **3,** 117–9.

6.35. TAYLOR, K.J.W., CARPENTER, D.A. and MCCREADY, V.R. (1973). Gray-scale echography in the diagnosis of intrahepatic disease. *J. clin. Ultrasound,* **1,** 284–8.

6.36. TAYLOR, K.J.W., CARPENTER, D.A. and MCCREADY, V.R. (1974). Ultrasound and scintigraphy in the differential diagnosis of obstructive jaundice. *J. clin. Ultrasound,* **2,** 105–16.

6.37. TAYLOR, K.J.W. and HILL, C.R. (1975). Scanning techniques in gray-scale ultrasonography. *Br. J. Radiol.,* **48,** 918–20.

6.38. TAYLOR, K.J.W. and MCCREADY, V.R. (1976). A clinical evaluation of gray-scale ultrasonography. *Br. J. Radiol.,* **49,** 244–52.

6.39. TAYLOR, K.J.W. and MILAN, J. (1976). Differential diagnosis of chronic splenomegaly: clinical observations and digital A-scan analysis. *Br. J. Radiol.,* **49,** 519–25.

6.40. TAYLOR, K.J.W. (1975). *Gray-scale Ultrasonography in the Investigation of Hepatobiliary Disease and Chronic Splenomegaly.* M.D. Thesis, University of London.

6.41. WANG, H.F., WANG, C.E., CHANG, C.P., KAO, J.Y., YU, L. and CHIANG, Y.N. (1964). The application and value of ultrasonic diagnosis of liver abscesses: a report of 218 cases. *Chin. med. J.,* **83,** 133–40.

6.42. WEILL, F., BOURGOIN, A., AUCANT, D., EISENCHER, A., FAIVRE, M., and GILLET, M. (1974). L'exploration tomo-echographique des dilatations de la voie biliare principale. *Arch. Fr. app. Dig.,* **63,** 453–72.

7. Ultrasonic investigation of the heart

F.G.M. ROSS

7.1. INTRODUCTION

Echocardiography* was introduced by Edler and Hertz [7.11] in 1954. They showed that various structures within the heart reflect ultrasound and that echoes can be obtained from the heart within the intact thorax. They presumed that the tracing obtained in patients with mitral stenosis originated from the anterior wall of the left atrium. This view was shared by others, but in 1961 Edler [7.8] showed that echoes could actually be obtained from the surfaces of the mitral, aortic and tricuspid valves. The method was subsequently developed fairly widely in the study of patients suffering from mitral valve lesions [7.10], largely because this was by far the easiest structure to locate and examine ultrasonically. Soon the method was shown to be a clinically useful technique for the detection of pericardial effusion [7.36]. Subsequently the use of echocardiography has been expanded greatly to include the examination of the walls of the heart, as well as the valves, and thus to extend its value into the assessment of cardiac function.

It is possible to make positive identification of several important echo sources within the heart by using a method [7.19] which depends on the injection of an ultrasonic contrast medium during catheterization of the various cardiac chambers. This injection produces cavitation in the blood at the tip of the catheter and the tiny bubbles which result are easily detectable by ultrasound. This ingenious technique has been further developed to allow the detection of intracardiac shunts [7.42].

7.2. ANATOMY

The front of the heart is normally covered by the lungs and pleura, except for a small triangular area in the left parasternal region extending down from the third or fourth costal cartilage. If the ultrasonic probe is placed over this 'bare' area, and between two costal cartilages or ribs, the ultrasound beam passes backwards in succession through the skin, the subcutaneous fatty tissue, the intercostal muscles, the two layers of the pericardium, the anterior wall of the heart, the cavity of the right ventricle, the anterior cusp of the mitral valve, the orifice of the mitral valve, the cavity of the left atrium and its posterior wall, and finally, the two layers of the pericardium posteriorly. Fairly frequently, the beam enters the left ventricular cavity by traversing the interventricular septum directly without

---

*Examination of the heart by pulse-echo ultrasound is known either as *echocardiography* or *ultrasoundcardiography*. The former term has been adopted by the American Institute of Ultrasound in Medicine [7.13] for this important examination and it is the term now almost exclusively used.

first passing through the right ventricular cavity. The exact anatomical course taken by the ultrasonic beam depends on the orientation of the heart with respect to the position of the probe on the chest wall. Sometimes the heart is rotated around its vertical axis, usually as a result of individual chamber enlargement [7.4], and this must be borne in mind when performing echocardiography.

The mitral valve consists of an orifice surrounded by the annulus fibrosus, which is a ring of fibrous tissue. To this ring, the thin membranous valve cusps are attached by their bases. The largest is antero-medial in position, and the smallest, postero-lateral; there are also two very small cusps situated in the commissures between the larger cusps. Inserted near the free edge of the cusps are a series of fine cordlike structures (the chordae tendineae), which are attached at their other ends to two cone-shaped papillary muscles which project from the walls into the cavity of the left ventricle. Occasionally, in normal hearts the chordae are muscular, and the papillary muscle inserts directly into the valve cusps. The function of the chordae tendineae is to prevent the valve cusps from inverting into the left atrium during ventricular contraction.

Continuous with the mitral valve ring, but slightly above in front and to the right of it, is the aortic valve. It has right and left anterior (coronary) cusps and one posterior (non-coronary) cusp, which are not supported by chordae tendineae. The aorta extends upwards and to the right from the aortic valve. The posterior wall of the aorta is continuous with the anterior cusp of the mitral valve and the anterior wall of the aorta is continuous with the interventricular septum.

Below, to the right and in front of the mitral valve, is the tricuspid valve. It has an anterior, medial (septal) and one or two posterior cusps to which chordae tendineae are attached on its right ventricular side. The pulmonary valve which has one anterior and two posterior cusps is above to the left and in front of the aortic valve. Its cusps, like those of the aortic valve, are pocket-shaped and are not supported by chordae tendineae.

The interventricular septum separates the right ventricle, which is in front and to its right, from the left ventricle, which is posterior and to its left. The septum is inclined at an angle to the horizontal plane from behind forwards, and its angle of inclination differs in normal individuals and also in pathological conditions of the heart. The septum consists of thick muscle for most of its length but in the immediate sub-aortic region it is membranous.

The heart with the proximal parts of the aorta, pulmonary artery and superior

Table 7.1. Cardiac dimensions: normal adult values [7.13].

	Mean (mm)	Range (mm)
Right ventricle diameter (supine)	15	7—23
Left ventricular internal diameter	46	35—56
Left ventricular posterior wall thickness	9	7—11
Interventricular septum thickness	9	7—11
Left atrial diameter	29	19—40
Aortic root	27	20—37
Aortic valve opening	19	16—26

vena cava, is invested within the two layers of the pericardium. Normal measurements of these structures are given in Table 7.1.

7.3. THE ULTRASOUND EXAMINATION

7.3.a.   General

In order to avoid a fast heart rate, which may arise from anxiety, it is advisable to explain to the patient prior to the examination the procedure for obtaining the echocardiogram. It is important to emphasise that he will experience no discomfort at all, and generally to put the patient at his ease as much as possible. The faster the heart rate, the less likely it is that a good echocardiogram will be obtained; with very fast heart rates, satisfactory tracings cannot be obtained. Most examiners use the mitral valve echoes as a landmark from which the rest of the heart can be explored. Therefore it is best to begin by describing the examination of the mitral valve.

7.3.b.   Mitral valve

The patient lies comfortably on a couch inclined to elevate the shoulders at an angle of about 10−15°. Electrocardiograph leads are attached, so that a correlation can be obtained between the ECG and the echocardiogram. Sometimes it is also useful to fix a phonocardiograph microphone on to the chest. Some coupling liquid (liquid paraffin, olive oil, or proprietary gel) is smeared on the skin of the front of the chest, over the area to be used for the examination. The third intercostal space is palpated and the probe is positioned over it, 10 mm or so to the left of the sternal edge. The probe is held vertical to the skin surface or angulated slightly upwards and medially in a direction towards the right shoulder. It is then moved slowly laterally until an echo from the anterior cusp of the mitral valve is obtained. If the echo is not obtained from the third interspace, the space below it is explored in the same manner. Occasionally, the fifth interspace must be used. The mitral valve echo is usually obtained within 20 or 30 mm of the sternal edge. In patients with large hearts, however, it may be necessary to move the probe even more laterally. If the mitral valve echo is not obtained with the patient in the inclined position, the examination may succeed if the patient lies flat, or is rotated a little towards his left side. When the echo from the anterior cusp of the mitral valve has been picked up, the position of the probe is adjusted by angulating it through a few degrees either upwards or downwards, medially or laterally until the best quality trace (see Section 7.6) with the greatest amplitude of movement is obtained. The patient must breathe quietly during the examination. On occasions it is found that a good trace can be obtained only during the phase of expiration. The record of the examination must be made on these patients whilst the patient holds his breath on expiration. It is worth emphasizing that good echocardiograms of the mitral valve in young children can generally be obtained with considerable ease, provided that the child can be kept still. As the probe is moved on the anterior chest wall, the examiner watches the display. The position of the probe is adjusted until the echo from the anterior cusp of the mitral valve is identified by its kicking movement in a position about 60−80 mm deep in the otherwise echo-free space between the echoes from the interventricular septum in front and the left atrial or ventricular wall behind. Slight downward angulation or movement of the probe from the best recording position for the anterior cusp usually enables echoes from the mitral valve posterior cusp to be obtained. Strenuous efforts should be made to obtain echoes from the posterior cusp in all examinations.

7.3.c.   Aortic root and aortic valve

Echoes from the aortic root and aortic valve may be obtained by angulating the probe medially and a little towards the patient's head from the position in which the mitral valve echo has been obtained [7.19].

7.3.d.   Tricuspid valve

Echoes from the tricuspid valve may be picked up by angulating the probe downwards towards the patient's feet and to the right and anteriorly from the mitral valve recording position. Echoes from the tricuspid valve are most easily recorded in patients who have enlargement of the right side of the heart.

7.3.e.   Pulmonary valve

This is the most difficult valve to examine. It may be located by angulating the probe upwards and to the left from the aortic valve position [7.13].

7.3.f.   Interventricular septum

If the probe is angulated downwards towards the patient's feet from the position in which the echoes from mitral valve have been obtained, echoes from the anterior and posterior surfaces of the interventricular septum are obtained. If this manoeuvre fails with the patient lying on his back, it may be successful if the patient is rotated towards the left side. Moreover, rotation of the patient into this position may facilitate examination of the aortic and mitral valve.

7.3.g.   Posterior heart wall

The same manoeuvre as described for the interventricular septum also produces good echoes from the posterior wall of the left ventricle revealing its inner (endocardial) surface and outer (epicardial) surface behind which are echoes from the pericardium and lung. In order to measure the left ventricular diameter and the thicknesses of the septum and posterior wall of the left ventricle, a point is selected just at the inferior part of the mitral valve where echoes from the anterior cusp or chordae tendineae can still be recorded. The posterior wall of the left ventricle is identified by its forward movement in systole. Most frequently echoes from the posterior wall of the left atrium are obtained behind the mitral valve anterior cusp echo, particularly if the probe is angulated upwards from the mitral valve position. The posterior wall of the left atrium can be distinguished from that of the left ventricle because it moves posteriorly during systole and its amplitude of movement is relatively small.

7.3.h.   Arc scan of left heart

If the direction of the ultrasonic beam is slowly altered downwards and laterally from the position of the ascending aorta towards the apex of the heart whilst a slow continuous recording is made on a strip chart recorder, an echographic tracing of the movements of the various heart structures is recorded from base to apex [7.13]. This is particularly useful for showing the continuity, or lack of continuity, between the anterior and posterior aortic walls with the interventricular septum and the anterior cusp of the mitral valve respectively.

7.3.i. Right ventricle
In most echocardiographic examinations the strong proximal echoes include those arising from the anterior wall of the right ventricle, the right ventricular cavity and the septum. If they are suppressed when the transducer is in the position used to show the interventricular septum, the right ventricular cavity can be shown. This is easier to demonstrate when the right ventricle is enlarged.

7.3.j. Atrial septum
If the probe is placed over the fourth or fifth interspace to the right of the sternum and directed medially and towards the patient's head, echoes from the interatrial septum can be identified at a depth of 40—60 mm [7.19].

7.4. CAUSES OF FAILURE TO OBTAIN AN ECHOCARDIOGRAM OF THE MITRAL VALVE

The ultrasonic examination of the mitral valve, and therefore usually of the rest of the heart, fails in about 8 per cent of patients. Occasionally no explanation can be found for this but, in the majority, failure is due to one or more of the following abnormalities:

(i) *The chest wall*
Obesity is a frequent cause of failure of the examination. This is because in obese patients, particularly women with large breasts, it may be very difficult to apply and maintain the probe over an intercostal space and to avoid impinging the beam onto a rib. A similar situation may arise in obese men with large anterior chest muscles.

In some patients with a marked degree of sternal depression, which may be in association with some obesity, the shape of the thoracic cage and the consequent displacement of the heart leads to failure to obtain an echocardiogram. Similarly, after left-sided thoracotomy, particularly for mitral valvotomy, the intercostal spaces may be so distorted and narrowed that echocardiography proves to be impossible.

(ii) *The lungs*
In some normal people, the left lung entirely covers the heart anteriorly. In patients suffering from emphysema, the lung volume is increased and the left lung may expand to cover the front of the heart. In such patients, the air-containing lung in front of the heart prevents the penetration of the heart by the ultrasound beam.

(iii) *The heart*
In patients with fast heart rates (of more than 80 per minute), the valve cusp

movements may be so rapid that the interpretation of the echocardiogram may be very difficult, or even impossible.

7.5 NORMAL ECHOGRAPHIC APPEARANCES

The usual convention in time-position recordings (Section 2.1.i) of cardiac valve movements is for upward deflexions of the trace to correspond to movements of the valve structure towards the ultrasonic probe. Thus, in the case of the anterior cusp of the mitral valve, upward deflexion of the trace represents opening of the valve.

7.5.a. Mitral valve
Echocardiograms* obtained from individuals with normal mitral valves are shown in Fig. 7.1.

(i) *Anterior cusp*
During left atrial contraction, the mitral valve opens and the echocardiogram of the anterior cusp traverses an upward deflexion to point A (Fig. 7.2.a), which occurs just after the P wave of the electrocardiogram. This is followed by a rapid downstroke through point B to point C (Fig. 7.2.b), produced by left ventricular contraction closing the valve. Point C coincides with the first heart sound, and represents the position of maximum closure of the mitral valve. The $A-C$ slope is sometimes referred to as the '*systolic slope*'. Point C is followed by a slow rise of the trace to point D (Fig. 7.2.c), produced by the forward movement of the whole valve structure and its ring that occurs during ventricular systole. The first component of the second heart sound, which indicates the time of closure of the aortic valve, occurs $0.01-0.05$ s before point D. As the ventricle relaxes, the valve cusps swing wide open and the echocardiogram trace rises steeply upwards to point E, which represents the position of maximum opening of the valve (Fig. 7.2.d). As the ventricle fills rapidly with blood from the left atrium, the anterior cusp of the valve is forced backwards from the open position; in addition, as the muscle of the ventricular walls relaxes, the valve ring moves backwards. During this phase, the echocardiogram trace may transcribe a two-phase downward slope, sometimes referred to as the '*diastolic slope*', through point F_0 to point F (Fig. 7.2.e), the first part of the slope ($E-F_0$) being less steep than the second part (F_0-F). The $E-F$ slope may also be straight, however, the two phases being merged into one. After point F, the trace may remain level for a short period during the phase of slow ventricular filling, particularly if the heart rate is slow. Very occasionally, a low amplitude rise may be seen shortly after the point F, but more frequently the trace moves directly to the next A wave.

In young persons, sinus arrhythmia occurs as a normal variant in the heart rhythm. In this condition, the heart rate increases during inspiration and slows during expiration. On the echocardiogram, the A wave merges into the E wave as

*Three types of recordings are used to illustrate this chapter. The *photographic* recordings were made with an Eskoline 20 instrument; the *strip-chart* recordings were made with the same ultrasonic system and a Kent-Cambridge fibre-optic paper oscillograph; and the *analogue* recordings were made with a custom-built ultrasonic system and time-to-voltage analogue converter [7.47] and a Mingograf ink-jet paper oscillograph.

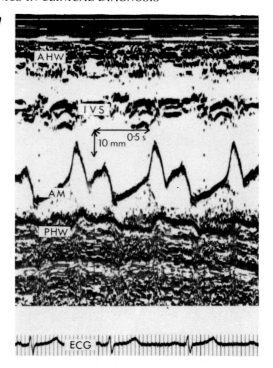

Fig. 7.1 Normal mitral valve echocardiograms. (*a*) Anterior cusp. (*b*) Anterior cusp, showing disappearance of A wave during inspiration. (*c*) Posterior cusp. *Key*—AHW: anterior heart wall; AM: anterior cusp of mitral valve; IVS: interventricular septum; PHW: posterior heart wall; PM: posterior cusp of mitral valve; ECG: electrocardiogram.

the heart rate quickens during inspiration, and then as the heart slows down during expiration, the *A* wave separates out again. Therefore, when the heart rate is fast, the echocardiogram is a single-peak trace; but at lower rates, it is a two-peak trace. Intermediates occur in which the *A* wave appears very shortly after the *E* wave and before the anterior cusp has had time to move any distance towards closure in early ventricular diastole. Similar variations in the appearances of the echocardiogram can be produced by other conditions which lead to variable *R*−*R* intervals.

(ii) *Posterior cusp*

The posterior cusp of the mitral valve is in contact with the anterior cusp during ventricular systole. The two cusps separate and move in opposite directions during diastole. The echo from the posterior mitral cusp transcribes a mirror image of the anterior cusp movement in diastole but it is of lower amplitude. The echoes from the two cusps merge during systole.

(iii) *Chordae tendineae*

Linear echoes arising from the chordae tendineae may be seen either in front of the anterior cusp, or behind the posterior cusp in systole. In the case of the anterior cusp they may produce several echoes parallel to those arising from the cusp.

b

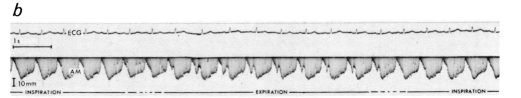

c

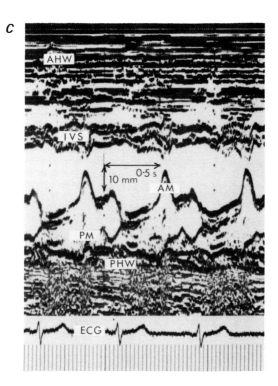

Note: The photographically recorded echocardiograms illustrating this Chapter (such as Figs. 7.1.*a* and 7.1.*c*) are marked by matrices of calibration dots: the horizontal dot spacing corresponds to 0.5 s, and the vertical, to 10 mm. The time scales, which are written at the bottoms of many of these recordings, correspond to 40 ms per division.

7.5.b. Aorta and aortic valve

The anterior and posterior walls of the ascending aorta move in directions parallel to each other, forwards during systole and early diastole and backwards during the remainder of diastole. An echocardiogram is shown in Fig. 7.3. In front of the aorta is the outflow tract of the right ventricle and behind it is the left atrium. The aortic valve cusps are seen as a linear echo in diastole, central in the aorta. In systole the right coronary cusp moves anteriorly and the left non-coronary cusp moves posteriorly, and their movements have a box-like pattern. Fine fluttering of the cusps in systole may be seen as a normal phenomenon.

7.5.c. Tricuspid valve

The movements of the cusps are similar to those described for the mitral valve.

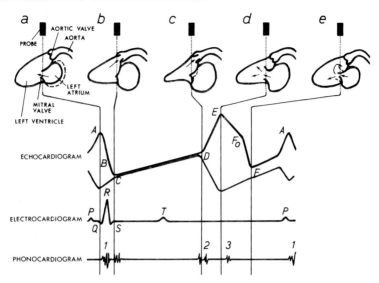

Fig. 7.2 Normal mitral valve echocardiogram, showing the time-relationships to the electrocardiogram and the phonocardiogram. The arrows indicate the directions of blood flow in the
diagrams of the left side of the heart. On the echocardiogram, increasing downward
deflexion of the trace corresponds to increasing depth of the anterior cusp of the valve (*i.e.*
closing of the valve). (*a*) Atrial systole. (*b*) Early ventricular systole. (*c*) Late ventricular
systole. (*d*) Ventricular diastole: rapid filling phase. (*e*) Late ventricular diastole.

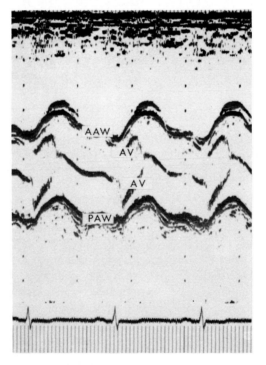

Fig. 7.3 Normal aortic valve echocardiogram. *Key*— AAW: anterior aortic wall; AV: aortic valve
cusp; PAW: posterior aortic wall.

7.5.d.   Pulmonary valve

This is the most difficult valve to examine, due to its orientation, and the clinical value of its echocardiogram has not yet been determined.

7.5.e.   Left ventricular walls

The posterior wall of the left ventricle and the interventricular septum move in opposite directions, approaching each other in systole and diverging in diastole. Various patterns of septal movement have been described in the normal individual [7.5].

7.6. QUALITY OF ECHOGRAPHIC RECORDING OF THE MITRAL VALVE

The form and quality of the echocardiographic trace depend to a considerable extent on the actual part of the valve cusp from which the ultrasound beam is reflected. This is illustrated in Fig. 7.4. If the ultrasound is reflected by the ring, a crescentic pattern is obtained; if it is reflected by the base of the cusp, a normal two-peaked trace is obtained, but it is of low amplitude in comparison with the

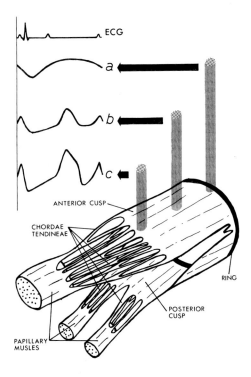

Fig. 7.4   Diagram illustrating the variation in the normal mitral valve echocardiogram according to the position at which the anterior cusp strikes the anterior cusp of the valve. (*a*) Reflexion from the ring. (*b*) Reflexion from a position approximately mid-way between the ring and the free edge of the cusp: echocardiogram has a normal shape, but a small amplitude and slope. (*c*) Reflexion from close to the free edge of the cusp: this is the correct echocardiogram.

trace which is obtained when the site of measurement is near the free edge of the cusp.

If the anterior cusp were to be a flat surface always moving at right angles to the direction of the ultrasound beam, good clear traces would generally be obtained because the echoes would be a fairly constant amplitude. The anterior cusp has a curved surface which may be irregular, however, and it oscillates backwards and forwards swinging on its attached peripheral edge. Therefore, normal incidence may not always be achieved, with the result that the echo may fail to return to the transducer. In this connexion, it has been shown [7.37] that the echo amplitude from a diseased mitral valve leaflet is less critically dependent upon angulation than that from a normal valve. On the other hand, the ultrasound beam may pass beyond the free edge of the cusp, and be reflected

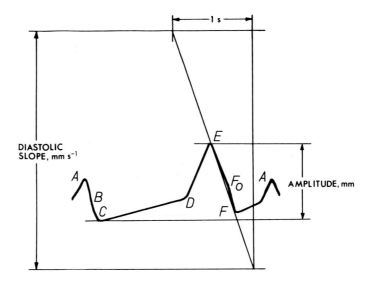

Fig. 7.5 Methods of measuring the amplitude of movement (*C* to *E*) of the anterior cusp of the mitral valve, and the speed of movement (the *diastolic slope*).

from a more posterior structure. In both of these cases, the echocardiographic recording is discontinuous, whether the recording is made by the photographic or by a continuous strip recorder method. It is very important for the accurate interpretation of echocardiographic traces that the occurrence of these phenomena should be recognized.

7.7. MEASUREMENTS FROM THE ECHOCARDIOGRAM

The evaluation of the echocardiographic recordings requires that they should be calibrated in terms of distance and time. Although some instruments are calibrated during manufacture, it is advisable that a periodic check should be made; a suitable calibrator is described elsewhere [7.47].

7.7.a.   Mitral valve

(i)   *Speed of movement*
The speed of movement of the valve cusp (sometimes referred to as the *slope* of the echocardiogram) at any phase of the cardiac cycle may be estimated by drawing a line parallel to the corresponding part of the echocardiogram, and then by measuring the distance between points on this line separated by 1 s. Usually, the speed of movement immediately following the point F_0 is estimated, as illustrated in Fig. 7.5. Typical values are given in Table 7.2. The speed of

Table 7.2. Mitral valve anterior cusp: speed and amplitude of movement.

	Diastolic slope $(mm\ s^{-1})$		Amplitude (mm)	
	Mean	Range	Mean	Range
Bristol series	114	70–160	22	14–33
King [7.25]		80–150		20–35
Layton et al. [7.26]	92	58–139		
Madeira et al. [7.30]	173	115–225		
Roger and Sumner [7.39]	176	128–234	29	22–41

movement of the valve is related to various clinical measurements; thus, in a series [7.20] of 24 patients with mitral stenosis, there was a statistical correlation with pulmonary arterial wedge pressure ($r = -0.66$) and with the mitral valve area estimated at operation ($r = 0.72$). If the valve movement is very restricted, however, the speed of movement is not a reliable index of stenosis [7.12].

(ii)   *Amplitude of movement*
The distance between points E and C (Fig. 7.5) represents not only the opening movement of the anterior cusp of the valve (which is approximately the distance between the points D and E), but also the forward movement of the whole valve structure, including the ring, which occurs as the result of the contraction of the ventricular muscle during systole. Typical values are given in Table 7.2.

(iii)   *Thickness of valve cusp*
An estimate of the thickness of the valve cusp may be made by inspection of the corresponding echo on an A-scope display, or on a suitable photographic or strip recorder time-position recording.

7.7.b.   Left ventricle
Valuable information in respect of the size and function of the left ventricle can be obtained from a measurement of its antero-posterior diameter (internal dimension) just distal to the level of the mitral valve. Normal values are listed in Table 7.1. The dimension is measured from the left side of the interventricular septum to the endocardial surface of the left ventricular posterior heart wall. The measurements are made at end-diastole (at the time of the Q wave of the

electrocardiograph) and at end-systole (at the time of the peak anterior movement of the posterior heart wall). The volume of the left ventricle can be calculated by cubing its internal diameter [7.14]. This calculation is shown to be valid so long as the long axis of the ventricle (apex to base) is equal to twice the short axis (antero-posterior diameter). As the ventricle enlarges in response to disease, the ratio of the long to the short diameters decreases and, therefore, the larger the ventricle, the greater the overestimation of the volume.

The *stroke volume* is calculated by subtracting the end-systolic volume from the end-diastolic volume. The *cardiac output* is calculated by multiplying the stroke volume by the heart rate. The *ejection fraction* is calculated by dividing the stroke volume by the diastolic volume.

7.7.c. Interventricular septum
The width of the interventricular septum is measured in end-diastole with the ultrasonic beam in the same position as is used to measure the internal diameter of the left ventricle. The range of the normal dimension is given in Table 7.1.

7.7.d. Posterior heart wall
The posterior heart wall consists of the left atrium superiorly and the left ventricle inferiorly, the mitral valve dividing the two. Echocardiographically, they can be easily distinguished because the left ventricular posterior wall moves forwards during systole, whereas the left atrial posterior wall moves backwards during ventricular systole. The inner endocardial surface of the left ventricular posterior wall can be distinguished from the outer epicardial surface behind which are the echoes from the lung. Just anterior to the endocardial surface, echoes may be obtained from the chordae to the posterior cusp of the mitral valve and these must be distinguished from the endocardial echo. The thickness of the left ventricular posterior wall can be measured from its endocardial to its epicardial surfaces. Normal values are given in Table 7.1. From measurements of the thickness of the ventricular wall, and also of the diameter of the ventricle, estimations of the total left ventricular mass can be made. Echocardiography has been used to determine the mean and peak velocities of the posterior wall motion as a measurement of left ventricular contractility. Another estimate of left ventricular function may be made echocardiographically by calculating the mean velocity of circumferential fibre shortening of the left ventricle [7.32].

7.7.e. Right ventricle
The distance between the anterior wall of the right ventricle and the right side of the interventricular septum can be measured from echocardiographic recordings. Careful adjustment of the swept gain is necessary to obtain satisfactory results. The measurement gives an estimate of the size of the right ventricular cavity. The thickness of the right ventricular wall can also be measured. Normal values are given in Table 7.1.

7.7.f. Aorta
The diameter of the root of the aorta is measured from the outer margin of the anterior wall to the inner aspect of the posterior wall. It varies slightly between

end-systole and end-diastole: normal values are given in Table 7.1. The distance separating the cusps of the aortic valve during systole can be measured and also the distance of the cusp echoes during diastole from the anterior and posterior walls. Eccentricity of the echo from the aortic valve cusps in diastole in a valuable sign of the presence of bicuspid aortic valve.

7.7.g. Left atrium
The antero-posterior diameter of the left atrium is measured at the level of the aortic root, from the anterior surface of the posterior aortic wall to the anterior surface of the left atrial posterior wall at end-systole. Normal values are given in Table 7.1.

7.7.h. Pulmonary artery
No useful measurement of the pulmonary artery can be made in adults. In infants, on the other hand, the two walls of the pulmonary artery can be demonstrated and the distance between them can be measured. Hence, the ratio of the widths of the pulmonary artery to the aortic root can be calculated. This can be helpful in the diagnosis of certain congenital heart lesions.

7.8   THE MITRAL VALVE ECHOCARDIOGRAM IN DISEASE
The most common abnormalities of the mitral valve are due to previous rheumatic fever. This can result in narrowing (or stenosis) of the valve, regurgitation, or a combination of stenosis and regurgitation, one or the other being dominant. The speeds and amplitudes of the mitral valve cusp in various clinical conditions are given in Table 7.3.

7.8.a.   Mitral stenosis
In mitral stenosis, there is obstruction to the flow of the blood from the left atrium to the left ventricle, due to narrowing of the valve orifice. The cusps may be thickened by fibrosis. There may be fusion of the commissures and calcification in the cusps as well as in the valve ring. In addition, the chordae tendineae

Table 7.3. Speed and amplitude of movement of the anterior cusp of the mitral valve in various clinical conditions (Bristol series).

Clinical condition	Number of patients	Diastolic slope (mm s^{-1})		Amplitude (mm)	
		Mean	Range	Mean	Range
Stenosis	157	19	6–40	17	8–32
Regurgitation					
All cases	50	75	10–280	22	10–55
Pure	13	198	120–280	33	22–55
Mixed stenosis and regurgitation					
Dominant stenosis	30	20	10–36	16	10–22
Dominant regurgitation	7	77	55–90	24	20–30

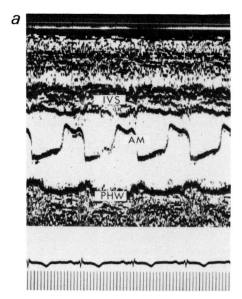

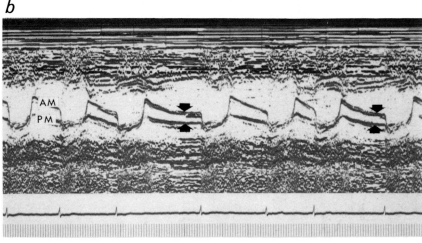

Fig. 7.6 Echocardiograms showing mitral stenosis. (*a*) Normal rhythm. (*b*) Atrial fibrillation: two long R-R intervals are shown (arrowed), in which both cusps are virtually stationary towards the end of the intervals. (*c*) Atrial fibrillation: multiple *A* waves (arrowed).

are shortened and thickened. As the obstruction increases, the pressure in the left atrium rises in order to maintain the cardiac output. The rapid backward motion of the anterior cusp (which normally occurs during early diastole) cannot take place in the presence of mitral stenosis because the raised left atrial pressure and the rigidity of the valve cusps result in a slow filling rate of the ventricle. Consequently, the backward motion of the anterior cusp is slower, but it continues for a longer time, than that of the normal valve. Therefore, in these patients, the normal rapid $E-F$ diastolic slope of the echocardiogram is replaced by a more gradual slope, which continues throughout diastole to the next wave if the patient is in normal rhythm. This is illustrated in Fig. 7.6.a. If the patient is in

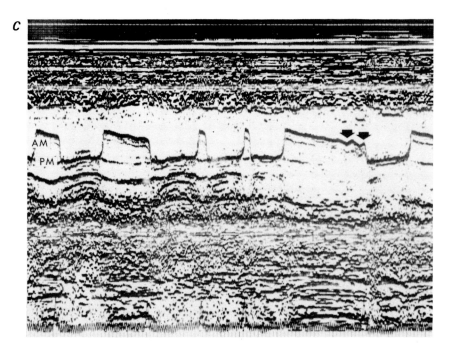

atrial fibrillation, however, the *A* wave is frequently absent, and the diastolic slope continues to point *B* on the systolic slope (Fig. 7.6.b and c). It has been observed in some patients with mitral stenosis and atrial fibrillation that, if the *A* wave is absent when the interval between cardiac contractions is short, it may appear when this interval is longer. Occasionally, multiple *A* waves (up to about eight) may appear when the interval between contractions is long (Fig. 7.6.c). This indicates that the mitral valve cusps may oscillate towards opening in diastole in atrial fibrillation. It is interesting to note that the gradients of the diastolic slope in patients with mitral stenosis and atrial fibrillation are similar whether the interval is short or long, except that when the interval is very long the tracing may show an almost straight horizontal line during the later stage of diastole (Fig. 7.6.b). It is important that the transducer be so positioned that the echo from the posterior cusp is shown. In organic mitral stenosis, the posterior cusp tracing moves parallel to that of the anterior cusp in diastole [7.27]; this distinguishes the condition from other abnormalities in which the mitral valve is normal but the filling rate of the left ventricle is slow. Moreover, if the cusps are calcified, the echoes from them are correspondingly extended. A few instances of inorganic mitral stenosis are now being reported, however, in which the posterior cusp moves backwards in diastole. In such cases there are usually additional signs of inorganic disease; for example, the *A* wave may be reduced or absent, and there may be thickening of the anterior cusp [7.16, 7.27].

7.8.b.   Mitral regurgitation

Mitral regurgitation may be due to dilatation of the valve ring such as may occur in left heart failure, to disease of the cusps, which occurs in rheumatic heart

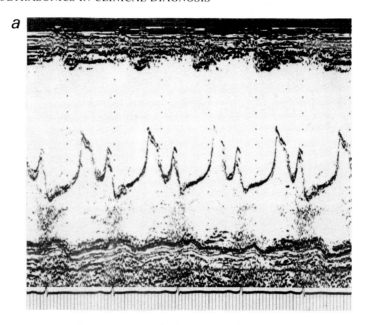

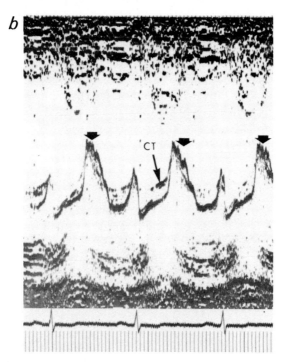

Fig. 7.7 Echocardiograms showing mitral regurgitation. (*a*) Pure rheumatic mitral regurgitation: the left ventricular outflow tract is large (80 mm diameter), the amplitude of movement of the anterior cusp is 38 mm, and its diastolic slope is 400 mm s^{-1}. (*b*) Ruptured chordae tendineae to the anterior cusp: there is oscillation of the cusp during the rapid filling phase of ventricular diastole (arrowed). *Key*—CT: chordae tendineae.

disease, or to disease of the chordae tendineae, such as rupture. When the valve ring is dilated, the movement of the anterior cusp may be normal, so that the corresponding echocardiogram is normal. In most cases of disease affecting the cusps, the echocardiogram is normal. In others the pattern of the echocardiogram is normal but the $E-F$ slope tends to be much more rapid than in normal individuals and the amplitude of the movement is usually increased [7.41]: see Table 7.3 and Fig. 7.7.a. A similar pattern may be seen in patients with a high flow rate through the mitral valve, which may occur in congenital heart disease with left to right shunt, such as ventricular septal defect or patent ductus arteriosus. Two conditions which cause mitral regurgitation can be diagnosed by echocardiography. They are prolapse of the posterior cusp of the mitral valve [7.6], and rupture of the chordae tendineae, either to the anterior or posterior cusp [7.7, 7.45]: this latter condition is illustrated in Fig. 7.7.b.

7.8.c. Combined mitral stenosis and regurgitation

In patients who have combined mitral stenosis and regurgitation, the shape of the echocardiogram pattern depends upon which of the lesions is dominant. If the cusps are rigid and with shortened chordae, producing dominant stenosis, the echocardiogram pattern is that of mitral stenosis. In patients with dominant regurgitation, the cusps are usually more mobile. The anterior cusp moves backwards fairly rapidly in early diastole, but the sustained left atrial pressure slows down this backward movement for the remainder of diastole [7.40], as in patients with pure mitral stenosis. On echocardiography there is a rapid early diastolic slope representing a cusp speed of movement of more than about

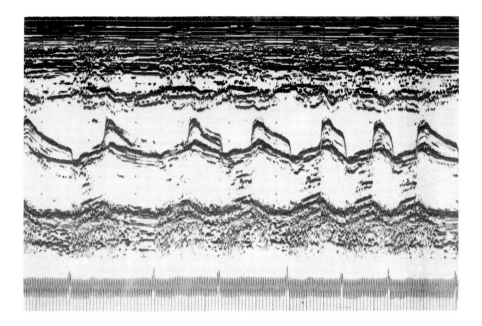

Fig. 7.8 Echocardiogram showing mixed mitral stenosis and regurgitation, with dominant regurgitation.

60 mm s^{-1} followed by a much more gradual slope which continues for the remainder of diastole (see Fig. 7.8 and Table 7.3).

7.8.d.   Cardiomyopathy

Hypertrophic obstructive cardiomyopathy is a condition in which there is asymmetrical hypertrophy of the interventricular septum and the wall of the left ventricle, together with obstruction during systole of the outflow tract of the ventricle. There is evidence that the obstruction is produced by abnormal forward movement of the anterior cusp of the mitral valve approaching the interventricular septum during systole, and that this results from changes in papillary muscle function. The same mechanism would also explain the mitral regurgitation that may be demonstrated in these patients by angiocardiography. On echocardiography [7.35, 7.43], the normal gradual anterior systolic movement (from position C to D) of the anterior cusp is replaced by a localized systolic anterior movement, which begins after the onset of ejection from the ventricle and continues to the later part of systole when the cusp returns to the position of closure. In addition, there is a reduced E–F diastolic slope, similar to that seen in mitral stenosis, but in hypertrophic obstructive cardiomyopathy it is due to the reduced rate of ventricular filling resulting from the low compliance of the

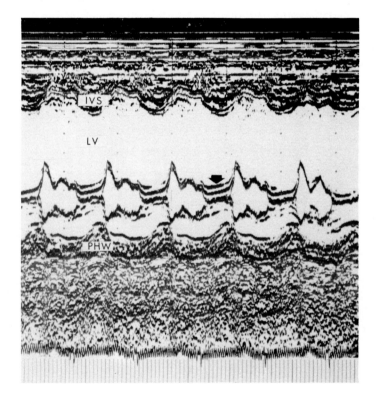

Fig. 7.9 Echocardiogram of mitral valve in a patient with severe coronary artery disease. The left ventricular cavity (LV) is large. The mitral valve cusps move normally. Multiple echoes are received from the chordae tendineae (arrowed).

ventricle. The latter may be seen in other conditions which produce massive left ventricular hypertrophy in the absence of outflow obstruction. The echocardiogram may demonstrate that the anterior mitral valve cusp comes into apposition with the interventricular septum during systole, and also in diastole at point E. There is also hypertrophy of the walls of the left ventricle but this is asymmetrical, the septum being relatively thicker than the posterior wall of the left ventricle. The ratio of the thickness of the septum to that of the posterior left ventricular wall is increased from the normal value of 1·0–1·6 to 1·6 – 3·0 [7.1].

In patients with congestive cardiomyopathy, and in some patients with coronary artery disease, the left ventricle is large and its walls may contract poorly. The large left ventricular cavity can be demonstrated by echocardiography. The mitral valve is equally easily demonstrated, and appears to be more posterior in position than in the normal. The pattern of the movement of its cusps is normal, but may be reduced in amplitude. Echoes from the chordae tendineae are also usually easily obtained. The features are illustrated in Fig. 7.9.

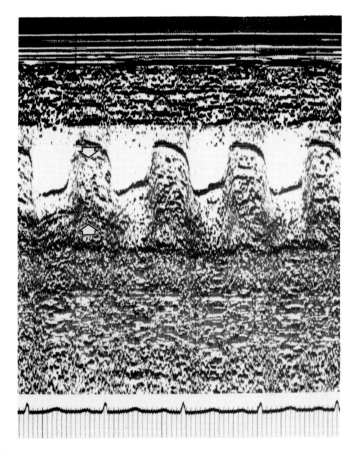

Fig. 7.10   Echocardiogram of mitral valve in a patient with left atrial myxoma. The diastolic slope is very low. Multiple echoes arising from the tumour (arrowed) are seen behind the anterior cusp in diastole.

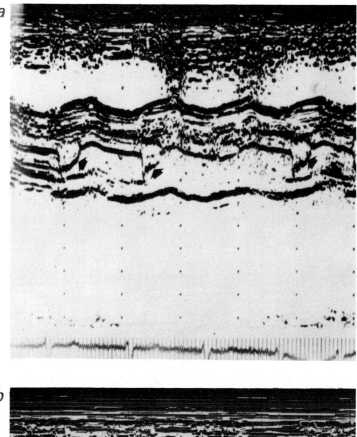

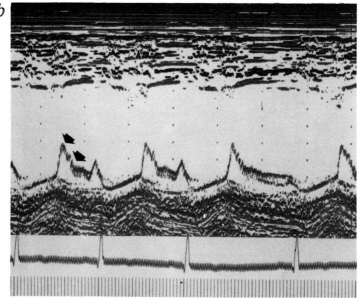

Fig. 7.11 Echocardiograms in aortic valve disease. (*a*) Aortic valve echocardiogram in calcific aortic stenosis. Dense echoes from the calcified valve cusps are shown within the aorta. The cusps open for a short time (arrowed) in systole. (*b*) Mitral valve echocardiogram in aortic regurgitation. Fluttering of the anterior cusp in diastole (arrowed) is clearly shown.

7.8.e. Left atrial myxoma

A myxoma of the left atrium is a pedunculated soft tissue tumour which arises from the interatrial septum. It may enlarge to such an extent that it herniates into the mitral valve orifice during ventricular diastole, so that part of the tumour is in the left ventricle, and part is in the left atrium and behind the anterior cusp of the mitral valve. During ventricular systole the tumour moves back into the left atrium. The tumour can be diagnosed by echocardiography because it gives rise to multiple echoes within the left atrium, and it may interfere with the movement of the anterior cusp of the mitral valve, particularly in diastole, producing a trace similar to that of mitral stenosis [7.9, 7.10]. A typical echocardiogram is shown in Fig. 7.10. Echocardiography is a very accurate method of detecting left atrial myxoma, and it should be used to screen patients who have unexplained systemic emboli.

7.9. AORTIC VALVE DISEASE

In patients with aortic stenosis, the excursion of the cusps is reduced, and if the cusps are calcified the echoes arising from them are extended (see Fig. 7.11.a).

In aortic regurgitation, no abnormality of the aortic valve cusps may be shown. In patients with aortic regurgitation and Austin-Flint murmur, however, the regurgitant jet of blood from the aortic valve in diastole, together with the blood flow through the mitral valve, produces fluttering of the anterior cusp of the mitral valve. This is illustrated in Fig. 7.11.b. The diastolic closure rate of the anterior cusp of the mitral valve is also usually reduced. In addition there may be early closure of the mitral valve due to the rapid rise in left ventricular pressure which prematurely reverses the gradient between the left ventricle and atrium.

Dilatation of the aorta and dissecting aneurysm can also be demonstrated [7.50].

7.10. TRICUSPID VALVE DISEASE

The tricuspid valve is difficult to demonstrate unless the right ventricle is enlarged. Tricuspid stenosis can be shown, and the pattern of the echocardiogram in this condition is similar to that of mitral stenosis.

7.11. PROSTHETIC VALVES

The movements of prostheses of the mitral and aortic valves can be studied by echocardiography [7.17, 7.48]. The approach to the aortic valve prosthesis is with the transducer in the suprasternal notch: it is difficult procedure [7.21]. The normal technique is used to demonstrate the mitral valve prosthesis. The pattern of the echocardiographic trace varies according to the type of prosthetic valve that is being used. An example of a Starr-Edwards valve in the mitral valve ring is shown in Fig. 7.12. Disc valves such as the Bjork-Shiley valve give a different pattern. Malfunction of the mitral valve prosthesis can also be detected [7.33, 7.34]

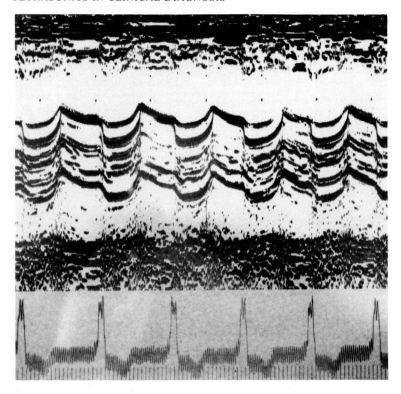

Fig. 7.12 Echocardiogram of unusually functioning Starr-Edwards prosthesis in the mitral position.
The multiple echoes arise from the ball and the cage.

7.12. PERICARDIAL EFFUSION

In normal individuals, the space between the two layers of pericardium investing
the heart is a potential space only, and on echocardiography it is not possible to
differentiate the echoes from the chest wall or the posterior pleura and the walls
of the heart. If fluid develops in the pericardial space, however, it may separate
the heart walls from the chest wall in front and the pleura behind, and these
structures can then be identified on echocardiography as separate echoes,
because the space where the intervening pericardial fluid has collected is echo-
free (see Fig. 7.13). Ultrasound provides a quick, safe and fairly reliable method
of detecting or excluding pericardial effusion [7.15, 7.36].

7.13. STUDIES USING INTRACARDIAC PROBES

Small transducers mounted on catheters have been used for the demonstration
and evaluation of atrial septal defects [7.31].

7.14. CROSS-SECTIONAL CARDIAC IMAGING

In order to visualize cardiac structure and function better, systems which display
two-dimensional cross-sections of the heart have been developed. This may be

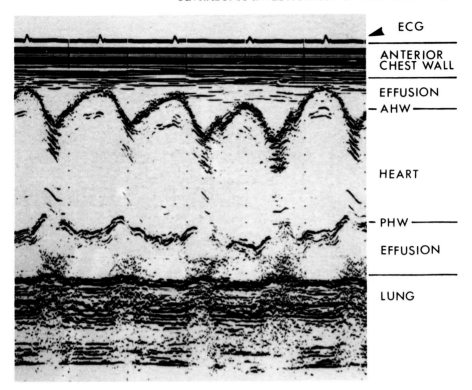

Fig. 7.13 Echocardiogram showing the regions between the anterior chest wall and the pleura posterior to the heart, demonstrating pericardial effusion.

achieved by the use of B-scanning techniques either of the real-time or of the ECG-triggered type (see Section 2.1.e). The latter shows a cross-section at a predetermined phase in the cardiac cycle, such as end-diastole. This method has many disadvantages including inability to produce dynamic studies. Real-time cross-sectional imaging is necessary to overcome most of the difficulties. In one instrument [7.3], the probe contains 20 transducer elements in a linear array 80 mm long and 10 mm wide. Each element in sequence transmits a short ultrasonic pulse, and the echoes which it receives are displayed on the horizontal axis of the oscilloscope. The echoes from each element are displayed in the vertical axis of the oscilloscope according to their respective positions in the transducer. By fast electronic switching from one element to the other, a cross-section of the heart is explored and instantaneous images obtained at the rate of switching. Recording may be made on cinématograph film or video-tape through a television camera to produce a moving image. Interesting clinical findings have been described using this method [7.38].

7.15. CONGENITAL HEART DISEASE

Infants and young children are very suitable for examination by echocardiography because the ultrasonic beam passes through the cartilaginous sternum and ribs with little attenuation, so that the heart is usually more accessible than in adults. On the other hand, co-operation may be difficult to achieve and tachycardia, which alters the pattern of the echo trace, is frequently present. The normal echocardiographic findings in neonates have been well described [7.44]. Echocardiography is of value in the diagnosis of atrial septal defect (see Fig.

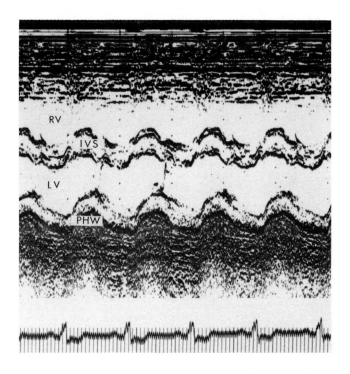

Fig. 7.14   Echocardiogram of left ventricle of a patient with large atrial septal defect. The interventricular septum and posterior heart wall move synchronously, indicating volume overload of the right ventricle (RV).

7.14), endocardial cushion defects, Fallot's tetralogy, double outlet right ventricle, congenital mitral stenosis, and many other conditions [7.18]. On occasions it may save the neonate from being subjected to cardiac catheterization, such as in the left heart syndrome, but more frequently it provides information that complements that obtained by cardiac catheterization and angiocardiography.

7.16.   DOPPLER TECHNIQUES IN THE STUDY OF THE HEART

Blood flow in the aortic arch can be detected by means of a Doppler transducer positioned in the suprasternal notch [7.29]. The correlations between velocity measurements made by this method, and various aspects of cardiac function, are quite encouraging [7.28]. Another potentially valuable technique, which gives information about the right heart and atrial septal defects, depends on the detection of disturbances in the jugular venous flow pattern [7.24] (see Section 9.1.b).

Doppler systems have been used for the detection and timing of the operations of the heart valves [7.2, 7.49]. The timing of the valve movements is related to the clinical condition of the valve. The method is considerably more sensitive, and less subject to artifacts, than phonocardiography. Microphones used for phono-cardiography are not very directional, and they rely for their selectivity on being placed close to the structure which is being studied. On the other hand, the ultrasonic beam of a Doppler system is highly directional, and so (within the limitation of transmission through ribs and lung) the structure being studied can be located with precision. Experiments have shown that signals from moving cardiac structures spaced along the beam can be separated by range-gating [7.46]. Recently, a trans-septal approach has been used to place a directional Doppler ultrasonic catheter tip velocimeter at the site of the mitral valve ring to study mitral flow velocity curves in the normal [7.22] and abnormal [7.23] valve. It is claimed that this is a reliable method for establishing the diagnosis (stenosis, regurgitation or a combination of these) and grading the severity of the lesion. It also provides a new approach to the understanding of haemodynamic distur-bances of the mitral valve on a beat-to-beat basis.

7.17.   SUMMARY

The principal applications of echocardiography are summarised in Table 7.4.

Table 7.4. Principal applications of echocardiography.

Detection and assessment of severity of mitral stenosis
Estimation of mobility and consistency of anterior cusp of mitral valve
Assessment of result of mitral valvotomy
Follow-up to assess progress of mitral stenosis and after mitral valvotomy
Assessment of dominance of stenosis or regurgitation in mixed mitral valve lesions
Detection and determination of cause of mitral regurgitation
Determination of presence or absence of mitral stenosis in patients with aortic valve disease (Austin-Flint murmur)
Detection of aortic regurgitation
Diagnosis of atrial myxoma, especially in the left atirum
Diagnosis of cardiomyopathy
Valve prosthesis studies, especially of the mitral valve
Estimation of left ventricular function
Diagnosis of pericardial effusion
Investigation of congenital heart disease, particularly right ventricular volume overload, left heart syndrome, and double outlet right ventricle

REFERENCES

7.1.   ABBASI, A.A., MACALPIN, R.N., EBER, L.M. and PEARCE, M.L. (1973). Left ventricular hypertrophy diagnosed by echocardiography. *New Eng. J. Med.,* **289**, 118–21.
7.2.   BELLET, S. and KOSTIS, J. (1968). Study of the cardiac arrhythmias by the ultrasonic Doppler method. *Circulation,* **38**, 721–36.
7.3.   BOM, N. (1962). *New Concepts in Echocardiography.* Leiden: Stenfert Kroese.
7.4.   CLELAND, W., GOODWIN, J., MCDONALD, L. and ROSS, D. (1969). *Medical and Surgical Cardiology.* Oxford: Blackwell.

7.5.   DIAMOND, M.A., DILLON J.R., HAINE, C.L., CHANG, S. and FEIGENBAUM, H.
       (1971). Echocardiographic features of atrial septal defect. *Circulation,* **43,** 129–35.
7.6.   DILLON, J.C., HAINE, C.L., CHANG, S. and FEIGENBAUM, H. (1971). Use of echocardi-
       ography in patients with prolapsed mitral valve. *Circulation,* **43,** 503–7.
7.7.   DUCHAK, J.M., CHANG, S. and FEIGENBAUM, H. (1972). Echocardiographic features of
       torn chordae tendineae. *Am. J. Cardiol.,* **29,** 260.
7.8.   EDLER, I. (1961). Ultrasoundcardiography. *Acta med. scand.,* **170,** suppl. 370.
7.9.   EDLER, I. (1965). The diagnostic use of ultrasound in heart disease. In *Ultrasonic Energy,* Ed.
       E. Kelly, pp. 303–21. Urbana: University of Illinois Press.
7.10. EDLER, I. (1966). Mitral valve function studied by the ultrasonic echo method. In *Diagnostic
       Ultrasound,* Ed. C.C. Grossman, J.H..Holmes, C. Joyner and E.W. Purnell, pp. 198–228. New
       York: Plenum Press.
7.11. EDLER, I. and HERTZ, C.H. (1954). The use of the ultrasonic reflectoscope for the
       continuous recording of the movements of heart walls. *K. fysiogr. Sällsk. Lund Förh.,* **24,**
       40–58.
7.12. EFFERT, S. (1959). Der derzeitige Stand der Ultraschallkardiographie. *Arch. Kreislauf-
       forsch.,* **30,** 213–68.
7.13. FEIGENBAUM, H. (1972). *Echocardiography.* Philadelphia: Lea and Febiger.
7.14. FEIGENBAUM, H., WOLFE, S.B., POPP, R.L., HAINE, C.L. and DODGE, H.T. (1969).
       Correlation of ultrasound with angiocardiography in measuring left ventricular diastolic
       volume. *Am. J. Cardiol.,* **23,** 111.
7.15. FEIGENBAUM, H., ZAKY, A. and WALDHAUSEN, J.A. (1967). Use of reflected ultra-
       sound in detecting pericardial effusion. *Am. J. Cardiol.,* **19,** 84–90.
7.16. FLAHERTY, J.T., LIVENGOOD, S. and FORTUIN, N.J. (1975). Atypical posterior leaflet
       motion in echogram in mitral stenosis. *Am. J. Cardiol.,* **35,** 675–8.
7.17. GIMENEZ, J.L., WINTERS, W.L., DAVITA, J.C., CONNELL, J. and KLEIN, K.S. (1965).
       Dynamics of the Starr-Edwards ball valve prosthesis—a cinéfluorographic and ultrasonic
       study in human. *Am. J. med. Sci.* **250,** 652–7.
7.18. GODMAN, M.J., THAM, P. and LANGFORD-KIDD, R.S. (1974). Echocardiography in the
       evaluation of the cyanotic newborn infant. *Br. Heart. J.* **36,** 154–66.
7.19. GRAMIAK, R., SHAH, P.M. and KRAMER, D.H. (1969). Ultrasound cardiography:
       contrast studies in anatomy and function. *Radiology,* **92,** 939–48.
7.20. GUSTAFSON, A. (1967). Correlation between ultrasoundcardiography, hemodynamics and
       surgical findings in mitral stenosis. *Am. J. Cardiol.,* **19,** 32–41.
7.21. JOHNSON, M.L. (1975). Echocardiographic evaluation of prosthetic heart valves. In *Cardiac
       Ultrasound,* Ed. R. Gramiak and R.C. Waag, pp. 149–84. St. Louis: Mosby.
7.22. KALMANSON, D., BERNIER, A., VEYRATT, C., WITCHITZ, S., SAVIER, C.H. and
       CHICHE, P. (1975). Normal pattern and physiological significance of mitral valve flow
       velocity recorded using transseptal directional Doppler ultrasound catheterisation. *Br. Heart
       J.,* **37,** 249–56.
7.23. KALMANSON, D., VEYRATT, C., BERNIER, A., SAVIER, C.H., CHICHE, P. and
       WITCHITZ, S. (1975). Diagnosis and evaluation of mitral valve disease using transseptal
       Doppler ultrasound catheterization. *Br. Heart J.,* **37,** 257–71.
7.24. KALMANSON, D., VEYRATT, C., CHICHE, P. and WITCHITZ, S. (1974). Noninvasive
       diagnosis of right heart diseases and of left-to-right shunts using directional Doppler ultra-
       sound. In *Cardiovascular Applications of Ultrasound.* Ed. R.S. Reneman, pp. 361–70.
       Amsterdam: North-Holland.
7.25. KING, D.L. (1974) (Ed.) *Diagnostic Ultrasound.* St. Louis: Mosby.
7.26. LAYTON, C., GENT, G., PRIDIE, R., MACDONALD, A. and BRIGDEN, W. (1973).
       Diastolic closure rate of normal mitral valve. *Br. Heart J.,* **35,** 1066–74.
7.27. LEVISMAN, J.A., ABBASI, A.S. and PEARCE, M.L. (1975). Posterior mitral leaflet motion
       in mitral stenosis. *Circulation,* **51,** 511–4.
7.28. LIGHT, H. (1974). Initial evaluation of transcutaneous aortovelography—a new non-invasive
       technique for haemodynamic measurements in the major thoracic vessels. In *Cardiovascular
       Applications of Ultrasound,* Ed. R.S. Reneman, pp. 325–60. Amsterdam: North-Holland.
7.29. LIGHT, H. and CROSS, G. (1972). Cardiovascular data by transcutaneous aortovelography.
       In *Blood Flow Measurement,* Ed. C. Roberts, pp. 60–3. London: Sector.
7.30. MADIERA, H.C., ZIADY, G., OAKLEY, C.M. and PRIDIE, R.B. (1974). Echocardiogra-
       phic assessment of left ventricular load. *Br. Heart J.,* **36,** 1175–81.
7.31. OMOTO, R. (1967). Intracardiac scanning of the heart with the aid of ultrasonic intravenous
       probe. *Jap. Heart J.,* **8,** 569–81.
7.32. PARASKOS, J.A., GROSSMAN, W., SALTZ, S., DALEN, J.E. and DEXTER, L. (1971). A

non-invasive technique for the determination of velocity of circumferential fiber shortening in man. *Circulation Res.,* **29,** 610–5.

7.33. PFEIFER, J., GOLDSCHLAGER, N., SWEATMAN, T., GERBODE, F. and SELZER, A. (1972). Malfunction of mitral ball valve prosthesis due to thrombus: report of 2 cases with notes of early clinical diagnosis. *Am. J. Cardiol.* **29,** 95–9.

7.34. POPP, R.L. and CARMICHAEL, B.M. (1971). Cardiac echography in the diagnosis of prosthetic mitral valve malfunction. *Circulation,* **44,** suppl. II, 33.

7.35. POPP, R.L. and HARRISON, D.C. (1969). Ultrasound in the diagnosis and evaluation of idiopathic hypertrophic subaortic stenosis. *Circulation,* **40,** 905–14.

7.36. PRIDIE, R.B. and TURNBULL, T.A. (1968). Diagnosis of pericardial effusion by ultrasound. *Br. med. J.,* **3,** 356–7.

7.37. REID, J.M. (1966). A review of some basic limitations in ultrasonic diagnosis. In *Diagnostic Ultrasound,* Ed. C.C. Grossman, J.H. Holmes, C. Joyner and E.W. Purnell, pp. 1–12. New York: Plenum Press.

7.38. ROELANDT, J., KLOSTER, F.E., TEN CATE, F.J., VAN DORP., W.G., HONKOOP, J., BOM, N. and HUGENHOLTZ, P.G. (1974). Multidimensional echocardiography. An appraisal of its clinical usefulness. *Br. Heart J.,* **36,** 29–43.

7.39. ROGER, J.C. and SUMNER, D.J. (1975). Measurement of the diastolic closure rate of normal mitral valve. *Br. Heart J.,* **37,** 504–13.

7.40. SEGAL, B.L., LIKOFF, W. and KINGSLEY, B. (1967). Echocardiography. Clinical application in combined mitral stenosis and mitral regurgitation. *Am. J. Cardiol.,* **19,** 42–9.

7.41. SEGAL, B.L., LIKOFF, W. and KINGSLEY, B. (1967). Echocardiography. Clinical application in mitral regurgitation. *Am. J. Cardiol.,* **19,** 50–8.

7.42. SEWARD, J.B. TAJIK, A.J., SPANGLER, J.G. and RITTER, D.G. (1975). Echocardiographic contrast studies: initial experiences. *Mayo Clin. Proc.,* **50,** 163–92.

7.43. SHAH, P.M., GRAMIAK, R. and KRAMER, D.H. (1969). Ultrasound localization of left ventricular outflow obstruction in hypertrophic obstructive cardiomyopathy. *Circulation,* **40,** 3–11.

7.44. SOLINGER, R., ELBI, F. and MINHAS, K. (1973). Echocardiography in the normal neonate. *Circulation,* **47,** 108–18.

7.45. SWEATMAN, T.W., SELLER, A. and COHN, K. (1970). Echocardiographic diagnosis of ruptured chordae tendineae. *Am. J. Cardiol.,* **26,** 661–2.

7.46. WELLS, P.N.T. (1969). A range-gated ultrasonic Doppler system. *Med. biol. Engng.,* **7,** 641–52.

7.47. WELLS, P.N.T. and ROSS, F.G.M. (1969). A time-to-voltage analogue converter for ultrasonic cardiology. *Ultrasonics,* **7,** 171–6.

7.48. WINTERS, W.L. GIMENEZ, J. and SOLOFF, L.A. (1967). Clinical application of ultrasound in the analysis of prosthetic ball function. *Am. J. Cardiol.,* **19,** 97–107.

7.49. YOSHIDA, T., MORI, M., NIMURA, Y., HIKITA, G., TAKAGISHI, S., NAKANISHI, K. and SATOMURA, S. (1961). Analysis of heart motion with ultrasonic Doppler method, and its clinical application. *Jap. Heart J.,* **61,** 61–75.

7.50. YUSTE, P., AZA, V., MINGUEZ, I., CEREZO, L. and MARTINEZ-BORDIA, C. (1974). Dissecting aortic aneurysm diagnosed by echocardiography. *Br. Heart J.,* **36,** 111–2.

FOR FURTHER READING

FEIGENBAUM, H. (1972). *Echocardiography.* Philadelphia: Lea and Febiger.

GRAMIAK, R. and WAAG, R.C. (1975) (Eds.). *Cardiac Ultrasound.* St. Louis: Mosby.

GOLDBERG, S.J., ALLEN, H.D. and SAHN, D.J. (1975). *Pediatric and Adolescent Echocardiography.* Chicago: Year Book Medical Publishers.

JOYNER, C.R. (1974). *Ultrasound in the Diagnosis of Cardiopulmonary Disease.* Chicago: Year Book Medical Publishers.

RENEMAN, R.S. (1974) (Ed.). *Clinical Applications of Ultrasound.* Amsterdam: North-Holland.

8. Ultrasonic investigations in urology

F.G.M. ROSS

8.1. INTRODUCTION

In recent years ultrasonic examination of the urinary tract has established itself as a reliable method. It is, however, usually used to complement other diagnostic methods, particularly radiology and radioisotopes. Ultrasound has an advantage in that it is a non-invasive technique and, so far as the kidney is concerned, needs no preparation of the patient. A further advantage is that ultrasound examination does not depend on the quality of renal function.

Ultrasonic examination of the bladder and prostate has not yet reached the same stage of development as its application to the kidney. It is likely, however, that it will be used more widely in the assessment of bladder and prostatic lesions in the future [8.8].

8.2. KIDNEY

It is advisable that intravenous urography should be performed prior to the ultrasound examination and that the films should be available at the examination. This is because it is important for the success of the examination that the clinical problem should be defined and the position of the kidneys, in particular their obliquity relative to the long axis of the spine, should be plotted. This allows for the best orientation of the ultrasound scan plane to the axis of the kidney. It is also important to determine whether any abnormality shown ultrasonically correlates in size and position with the abnormality demonstrated radiologically.

The patient is usually examined in the prone position; but, by scanning through the liver, it is possible to visualize the right kidney, and sometimes also the left kidney. Except when scanning infants [8.12], direct contact B-scanning methods are more convenient than those employing water coupling.

The A-scope has been used to detect renal stones at operation [8.9, 8.18], to identify the depth and position of kidney prior to biopsy [8.4] and radioisotope studies, and to distinguish between cystic and solid lesions [8.6, 8.16], particularly when the position of the lesion has first been determined by two-dimensional scanning.

For contact B-scanning, longitudinal, transverse and oblique sections are made usually during inspiration, as this makes the kidneys more accessible to the ultrasonic beam by displacing them downwards below the costal margin. Lower pole lesions may be better shown on expiration. Useful transverse sections of both kidneys may be obtained by sector scanning through a lateral intercostal space [8.20].

Longitudinal scans are made parallel to the spine at serial intervals of 5 to 10 mm. It is convenient to start scanning at about 60 mm from the midline, as this level usually passes through the kidney. It is best to demonstrate the kidney in its full long axis, and therefore oblique scans are frequently more informative than longitudinal scans. Transverse scans are then performed, relating their levels to that of the iliac crest; this level is best determined from the longitudinal scan. If the patient has a lordotic spine, it is important to incline the scan plane slightly towards the patient's head in order to achieve good contact of the probe face with the skin. If the patient lies with a pillow under the abdomen, it tends to reduce the degree of lordosis and also makes it easier for him to breathe. A frequency of 2 or 2·5 MHz is generally used, and scans are made at both high and low sensitivities. It must be realized that there is a small proportion of patients (1—2 per cent) in whom it is not possible to obtain an examination of the kidneys, due either to obesity, overlying gas, or bone.

8.3. INDICATIONS FOR ULTRASONIC EXAMINATION OF THE KIDNEY

The position, size and shape of the kidneys can be shown, and the kidney volume can be calculated.

8.3.a.   Renal masses
Undoubtedly the most frequent use of ultrasound in clinical practice is to determine whether a renal mass shown at intravenous urography is a cyst or a tumour, and to indicate whether cyst puncture or urography is the more appropriate further examination to be performed. It is important to realize that right-sided renal lesions are easier to demonstrate than left-sided ones, that lower pole lesions are easier to demonstrate than upper pole lesions, and that large masses are easier to show than small ones. These considerations should be allowed for when assessing the statistical reliability of the method. Renal lesions of less than 20 mm in diameter, though they may be identified, cannot be differentiated as to their pathological nature.

8.3.b.   Renal failure
In patients with poor renal function, who do not produce a diagnostic intravenous urogram, determination of renal size and configuration can be of great importance [8.8]. A differential diagnosis between shrunken pyelonephritic kidneys and obstructive uropathy can easily be made.

8.3.c.   Unilateral non-functioning kidney
If intravenous urography shows unilateral excretion, ultrasound examination can quickly determine whether or not there is a kidney in the expected position on the affected side. It can also be shown whether the cause is a small contracted kidney, hydronephrosis, or tumour.

8.3.d.   Renal displacement
Displacement of a kidney can be caused by tumour, abscess, haematoma, urinoma, aneurysm, or splenic enlargement; ultrasound can be very helpful in

determining which of these conditions is present. The relationship of the kidney to an intra-abdominal mass, even if there is no renal displacement, can be readily shown and this may be very helpful in the differential diagnosis.

8.3.e. Bilateral renal enlargement

Polycystic kidneys may be difficult to diagnose radiologically for certain, particularly when renal function is reduced. They are readily shown by ultrasound.

8.3.f. Radiotherapy planning

Localization of the kidney by ultrasound, for purposes of radiotherapy, is a valuable aid to planning. The depth, size and position of the kidney can be determined.

8.3.g. Renal biopsy or puncture

The best site for renal biopsy, puncture of a renal mass, or nephrostomy, can be determined; and if a transducer with a central hole in it is used, the needle can be directed through it with great accuracy [8.7].

8.3.h. Pregnancy

It is undesirable to use x-radiation to investigate pregnant women, unless it is impossible to avoid it. Therefore, in these patients the use of ultrasound in the diagnosis of probable renal lesions can be a most valuable adjunct to clinical examination.

8.3.i. Renal transplants

Ultrasound examination has become a valuable aid in the follow-up of patients with renal transplants. It is free of hazard, and it is not necessary to puncture an artery. Therefore, it can be used serially to detect complications to which transplanted kidneys are subject, such as rejection, obstruction, and perinephric collections of urine, blood or pus [8.15].

8.3.j. Fetal kidney

The kidneys and bladder of the fetus can be shown *in utero*; and with the more extensive use of ultrasound in obstetrics, more cases of intrauterine renal abnormality are bound to be shown, such as polycystic disease [8.5].

8.4. NORMAL ULTRASONIC APPEARANCES OF THE KIDNEY

In longitudinal section, the kidney is oval in outline and its surface is smooth. A typical scan is shown in Fig. 8.1.a. The kidney is well-differentiated from the surrounding muscles and abdominal organs. The cortex is anechoic. The calices, pelvis and blood vessels are shown as a central group of high amplitude echoes. If the kidney is duplex, or if there is a long major calix to the upper group of calices, the central echoes due to the calices are divided into two groups, a small upper pole one and a larger lower pole group. If the section is taken lateral to the position of the calices, no central echo line is shown. Frequently the ribs produce

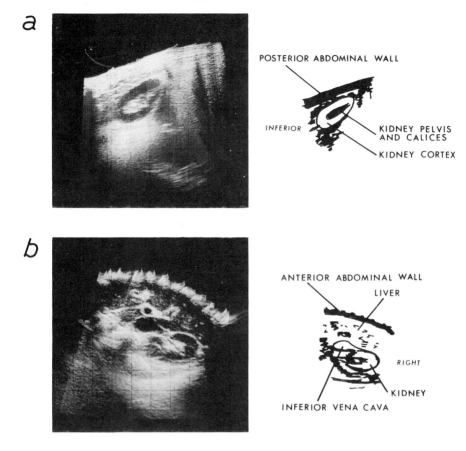

Fig. 8.1   Scans of normal kidney. (*a*) Posterior longitudinal scan, 70 mm right of midline. (*b*) Oblique transverse subcostal scan.

Note: With the exception of that in Fig. 8.5, the scans which illustrate this Chapter were made with a custom-built 2 MHz contact scanner.

linear 'shadows' across the upper part of the kidney. When scanned from the front in the supine position, it is important to note that the right kidney is oblique in position with its lower pole more anterior than the upper pole. In transverse sections, the kidney is oval or rounded, as illustrated in Fig. 8.1.b. The calices are seen as a rounded group of echoes nearly central if the section goes through one of the renal poles, or medially placed if the section goes through the renal pelvis. If the section is above or below the calices, the central echo group is absent. The ureters cannot be identified unless they are dilated.

8.5.   ULTRASONIC APPEARANCES IN KIDNEY DISEASE

8.5.a.   Renal carcinoma

Renal cell carcinoma, to be identified ultrasonically, must be large enough to produce deformity of the calices on intravenous urography. The usual clinical problem posed is the differential diagnosis of a renal space-occupying lesion shown on intravenous urography; but for purposes of description it is easier to detail the ultrasonic appearances of individual pathologies.

Fig. 8.2 is a scan showing a kidney tumour. Generally, the tumour indents displaces or destroys part of the central caliceal echoes. They are replaced by a mass which contain multiple random echoes at high gain. The mass bulges the outline of the kidney either locally along one surface, or produces diffuse enlargement of one pole. The outline of the mass is usually ill-defined. As the ultrasound beam passes through the mass it is attenuated so that the structures deep to the neoplasm are put into ultrasonic shadow, *i.e.* echoes arising deep to the neoplasm are of lower intensity than surrounding echoes. A characteristic of neoplasm is that the intensity of echoes arising within the lesion varies from place

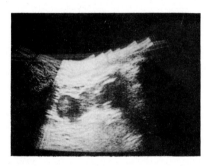
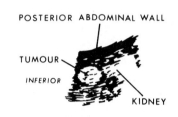

Fig. 8.2 Longitudinal scan 70 mm left of midline. The kidney is largely displaced out of the plane of the scan by a tumour of the lower pole.

to place, and therefore the echo pattern is uneven. Necrotic parts of the neoplasm have very low echogenicity whereas solid areas may be highly echogenic, *i.e.,* they may produce a complex echo pattern. An A-scan shows multiple echoes of varying amplitude throughout the mass. For example, in a group [8.19] of 30 patients with renal masses producing complex ultrasonic patterns, 18 (60 per cent) were carcinomata, 3 were renal abscesses, 2 were cysts with blood clot in them, and 1 each were caliceal cysts, simple cysts, localized polycystic disease, renal haematoma, ureteric obstructing tumour, renal sinus fat, and normal kidney.

8.5.b.   Renal cyst
Dependent on its size, a cyst produces indentation or displacement of the caliceal echoes, and a mass deforming the outline of the kidney. The mass may replace one or other pole, or it may extend out from the kidney surface. The outline of the mass is well-defined, particularly its deep surface which is shown as a fine crescentic white line. A typical scan is shown in Fig. 8.3. An A-scan shows no echoes arising within the mass. On the B-scan, as ultrasound is only slightly attenuated in the fluid in the cyst, there is an area of relatively higher intensity echoes deep to the cyst. At high gain settings, the cyst remains relatively anechoic compared with the surrounding structures, though some echoes scatter into it. For example, in a group [8.19] of 58 patients with suspected renal cysts, 56 (97

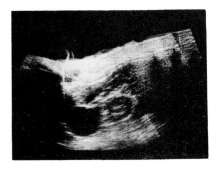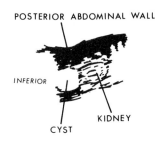

Fig. 8.3 Longitudinal scan 50 mm left of midline. There is a cyst, of about 40 mm diameter, involving the lower pole of the kidney.

per cent) were correctly diagnosed; one proved to be a renal carcinoma, and one, a renal abscess.

8.5.c. Polycystic disease

In polycystic disease, both kidneys are enlarged. The kidney outline may be lobulated, corresponding to the margins of the peripheral cysts on the surface. A typical scan is shown in Fig. 8.4. The normal central group of echoes from the calices is absent: it is replaced by multiple small fine echoes throughout the kidney, corresponding to the cyst walls. These echoes, separated by anechoic areas, may be close together if the cysts are small, but they may be quite far apart or there may even be circles of echoes if the cysts are larger. If polycystic kidneys are shown, the liver should be examined because hepatic polycystic disease may also be present. If multiple cysts are shown in only one kidney, multicystic disease is present.

8.5.d. Hydronephrosis

The kidney size depends on the type of hydronephrosis and its degree. In early pelvic hydronephrosis the central echoes are separated by the pelvic dilatation, producing a ring of echoes in the longitudinal section (see Fig. 8.5) and a crescent of echoes (C-sign) in the transverse section [8.3]. In more advanced pelvic

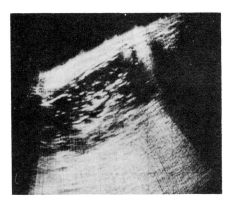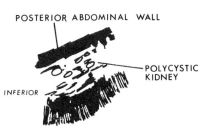

Fig. 8.4 Polycystic kidney disease. Longitudinal scan, 60 mm right of midline.

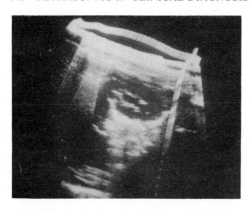
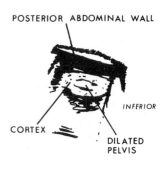

Fig. 8.5 Hydronephrosis associated with pregnancy. Longitudinal section, 50 mm left of midline.

Note: This scan was made with a Picker Echoview System 80L (see Appendix).

hydronephrosis, the dilated renal pelvis may be identified as a transonic mass medial to the kidney, and on occasions the upper part of the dilated ureter may be shown as a linear anechoic downward extension from the pelvis. In advanced hydronephrosis the calices are also dilated. In this event, the normal central echoes disappear and the kidney is enlarged. Coarse septa due to compressed renal tissue between the dilated and anechoic calices are demonstrated. Should a pelvic hydronephrosis become gross, and caliceal dilatation is not marked, then a large transonic mass is shown medial to the displaced kidney. If a large renal calculus is present in hydronephrosis it is shown as a group of dense echoes within the otherwise anechoic renal pelvis or calix, with ultrasonic shadowing beyond.

8.5.e.   Perinephric abscess
A perinephric abscess shows as an anechoic area adjacent to the intact kidney, and, if it displaces the kidney, this is most frequently in the forward direction.

8.6. THE BLADDER AND THE PROSTATE GLAND

For the demonstration of bladder and prostatic lesions, the bladder must be as full as possible. Longitudinal and transverse scans (with or without the transducer inclined towards the pelvis) are made.

8.6.a.   Bladder
It is possible to measure the distance between the anterior and posterior walls of the bladder using an A-scope [8.10, 8.11], but this information is inadequate for an accurate estimate to be made of the contained urinary volume. The method does have some clinical value, however, in revealing retained urine.

Although the volume of retained urine can be estimated by radiological methods, such investigations are undesirable, particularly in children, and they cannot be used repeatedly. The volume of the bladder may be estimated by serial two-dimensional transverse B-scans, however, using a planimeter to determine the area of the cross-section of the bladder in each scan plane. An average difference of 25 per cent was found in a comparison between ultrasonic and voided volume measurements in a series [8.11] of 26 patients. It seems that results of similar accuracy can be obtained more simply, however, using area estimates in a single transverse and a single longitudinal scan [8.1]. In 50 patients, the mean error using this method was 28 per cent, if the volume was greater than 100 ml. With smaller volumes, the ultrasonic estimate was very inaccurate.

Radiology and cystoscopy can be used to demonstrate most tumours of the bladder, but they have several disadvantages, such as x-ray hazard, risk of infection, and discomfort. Moreover, radiology is ineffective in poor renal function, and cystoscopy is especially difficult in stricture. Two-dimensional ultrasonic scanning readily demonstrates that the normal bladder, when filled with urine, is smooth in outline, pear-shaped in longitudinal section and with vertical lateral walls in transverse section. Intrinsic lesions of the bladder projecting into its lumen and extrinsic lesions pressing on the walls can be located by ultrasound examination of the fluid-filled bladder. A typical scan is shown in

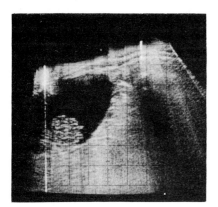 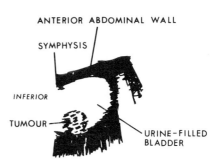

Fig. 8.6 Bladder tumour attached to posterior bladder wall, shown in longitudinal midline section.

Fig. 8.6. Tumours fungating into the bladder lumen can be demonstrated with considerable accuracy by radiology and can be seen and biopsied by cystoscopy. The contribution to management that ultrasound can make is to assess the presence or absence of wall infiltration, the length of the tumour base and the extent, if any, of infiltration into the pelvic soft tissues [8.2, 8.3]. Infiltration of the bladder wall is shown by increase in its thickness and lack of definition, together with deformity in advanced cases of the bladder outline. The response of the tumour to radiotherapy can be plotted by serial examination. The reliability with which these studies may be made is greatest when the bladder has a large capacity and the tumour is on the posterior wall. The lower part of the bladder behind the symphysis is anatomically rather inaccessible, but the rest of the anterior wall should be more clearly seen if a water-bath scanner were to be used.

8.6.b.   Prostate gland
The prostate gland is not readily accessible to conventional ultrasonic diagnostic

investigation, although if it is enlarged it can be seen protruding into the urine-filled bladder in scans made transcutaneously through the anterior abdominal wall [8.2]. Using this approach, the volume of the gland may be estimated [8.13, 8.22] and this can help the surgeon to choose between open surgery and transurethral resection.

An alternative method of visualizing the prostate depends on the use of a transrectal ultrasonic scanner [8.21]. Technically this is very attractive but it is aesthetically rather unacceptable to some patients, and the equipment is expensive.

8.7.   TESTIS

Direct contact scans of the testis, made transcutaneously through the scrotum, can reveal hydrocele, testicular abscess and tumour [8.14]. Torsion of the testis can be diagnosed by abnormal Doppler-shifted signals when the probe is held on the scrotum [8.17].

REFERENCES

8.1. ALFTAN, O. and MATTSON, T. (1969). Ultrasonic method of measuring urine. *Annls Chir. Gynaec. Fenn.*, **58**, 300–3.
8.2. BARNETT, E. and MORLEY, P. (1971). Ultrasound in the investigation of space-occupying lesions of the urinary tract. *Br. J. Radiol.*, **44**, 733–42.
8.3. BARNETT, E. and MORLEY, P. (1972). Diagnostic ultrasound in renal disease. *Br. med. Bull.*, **28**, 196–9.
8.4. BERLYNE, G.M. (1961). Ultrasonics in renal biopsy. An aid to determination of kidney position. *Lancet*, **2**, 750–1.
8.5. GARRETT, W.J., GRUNWALD, G. and ROBINSON, D.E. (1970). Prenatal diagnosis of fetal polycystic kidney by ultrasound. *Aust. N. Z. J. Obstet. Gynaec.*, **10**, 7–9.
8.6. GOLDBERG, B.B., OSTRUM, B.J. and ISARD, H.J. (1968). Nephrosonography: ultrasound differentiation of renal masses. *Radiology*, **90**, 1113–8.
8.7. GOLDBERG, B.B. and POLLACK, H.M. (1973). Ultrasonically guided renal cyst aspiration. *J. Urol.*, **109**, 5–7.
8.8. GREEN, W.L. and KING, D.L. (1976). Diagnostic ultrasound of the urinary tract. *J. clin. Ultrasound*, **4**, 55–64.
8.9. HEAP, G. (1968). Localization of urinary calculi by ultrasound. *Br. J. Urol.*, **40**, 485.
8.10. HOLMES, J.H. (1966). Ultrasonic studies of the bladder and kidney. In *Diagnostic Ultrasound*, Ed. C.C. Grossman, J.H. Holmes, C. Joyner and E.W. Purnell, pp. 465–80. New York: Plenum Press.
8.11. HOLMES, J.H. (1967). Ultrasonic studies of the bladder. *J. Urol.* **97**, 654–63.
8.12. LYONS, E.A., MURPHY, A.V. and ARNEIL, G.C. (1972). Sonar and its use in kidney disease in children. *Arch. Dis. Child.*, **47**, 777–86.
8.13. MILLER, S.S., GARVIE, W.H.H. and CHRISTIE, A.D. (1973). The evaluation of prostate size by ultrasonic scanning: a preliminary report. *Br. J. Urol.*, **45**, 187–91.
8.14. MISKIN, M. and BAIN, J. (1974). B-mode ultrasonic examination of the testes. *J. clin. Ultrasound*, **2**, 307–11.
8.15. MORLEY, P., BARNETT, E., BELL, P.R.F., BRIGGS, J.K., CALMAN, K.C., HAMILTON, D.N.H. and PATON, A.M: (1975). Ultrasound in the diagnosis of fluid collections following renal transplantation. *Clin. Radiol.*, **26**, 199–207.
8.16. OSTRUM, B.J., GOLDBERG, B.B. and ISARD, H.J. (1967). A-mode ultrasound differentiation of soft-tissue masses. *Radiology*, **88**, 745–9.
8.17. PEDERSEN, J.F., HOLM, H.H. and HALD, T. (1975). Torsion of the testis diagnosed by ultrasound. In *Ultrasound in Medicine*, Ed. D. White, p. 193. New York: Plenum Press.
8.18. SCHLEGAL, J.U., DIGGDON, P. and CUELLAR, J. (1961). The use of ultrasound for localising renal calculi. *J. Urol.*, **86**, 367–9.
8.19. SHERWOOD, T. (1975). Renal masses and ultrasound. *Br. med. J.*, **4**, 682–3.

8.20. TAYLOR, K.J.W. (1976). Gray-scale ultrasound B-scanning for assessment of the liver and the kidney. *Br. J. clin. Equipment*, **1**, 113–121.
8.21. WATANABE, H., KAIHO, H., TANAKA, M. and TERASAWA, Y. (1971). Diagnostic application of ultrasonotomography to the prostate. *Invest. Urol.*, **8**, 548–59.
8.22. WHITTINGHAM, T.A. and BISHOP, R. (1973). Ultrasonic estimation of the volume of the enlarged prostate. *Br. J. Radiol.*, **46**, 68–70.

9. Other ultrasonic investigations

F.G.M. ROSS AND P.N.T. WELLS

9.1. ANGIOLOGY

9.1.a. Angiography

Studies of the abdominal aorta have been made using A-scan [9.8, 9.21, 9.33], two-dimensional B-scan [9.2, 9.8, 9.10, 9.13, 9.14, 9.20, 9.21, 9.39] and time-position recording [9.8, 9.33] at frequencies in the range 1–3 MHz. The patient is examined in the supine position. Both direct-contact methods, and water-bath coupled two-dimensional scanning have been employed, although the former are generally the more convenient. Occasionally, it is impossible to visualize the aorta because of the intervention of intestines containing gas. In such circumstances, satisfactory results can sometimes be obtained later [9.21].

The examination is best begun by making a number of longitudinal two-dimensional B-scans parallel to, and extending as far as possible from the

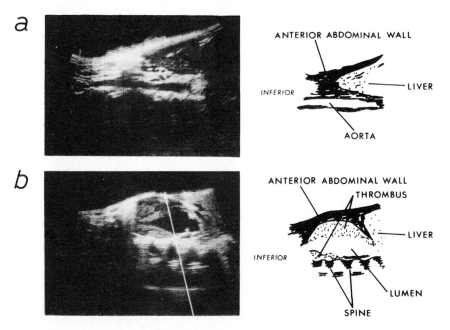

Fig. 9.1 Abdominal aorta, visualized in longitudinal midline sections. (*a*) Normal. (*b*) Aortic aneurysm: note thrombus and lumen.

Note: With the exception of that in Fig. 9.6, the scans which illustrate this Chapter were made with a custom-built 2 MHz contact scanner.

152

xiphoid to the symphysis. Typical scans are shown in Fig. 9.1. Sometimes, the tortuosity of the aorta precludes the visualization of its entire abdominal length in a single scan.

Although the diameter of the aneurysm can be estimated from the two-dimensional B-scan, this can more accurately be done from a time-position recording (in which the pulsations may help in the identification of the echoes from the walls of the aorta [9.8]), or from an A-scan in the case of a larger aneurysm with small pulsations [9.21]. Thus, in a series of 18 patients, the difference between operative or contrast aortographic measurements, and the ultrasonic estimates, did not exceed 6 mm. The demonstration of an aortic diameter of more than 30 mm is taken to be pathological [9.8].

Conventional radiological investigations of the aorta have several disadvantages. Calcification may allow the aorta to be visualized on a plain film. If this is not the case, aortography may be required. Ultrasonic scanning is useful in patients in whom aortography is contraindicated, and in serial examinations to detect changes in aortic size. A common clinical problem, in which ultrasonic examination can be helpful, is to determine whether a palpable pulsating abdominal mass is an aortic aneurysm or an anterior mass transmitting pulsations from a normal aorta behind it.

Although the aorta is the abdominal vessel which has received most attention in ultrasonic scanning, other arteries and veins can be demonstrated. It is generally possible to visualize the terminal position of the inferior vena cava by scanning through the liver [9.37], and in cases of IVC obstruction it may be possible either directly or indirectly to deduce the cause. The superior mesenteric and renal arteries, and the portal, superior mesenteric and renal veins, can also frequently be seen [9.22].

Pulse-echo techniques have also been used in evaluating aneurysms of the femoral artery [9.14], and in estimating the diameters of the thoracic aorta and the right pulmonary artery (with the ultrasonic probe in the suprasternal region) [9.12].

9.1.b.   Investigations of blood flow

(i)   *Blood flow in the placenta*
The use of the continuous wave Doppler method for the demonstration of the movements of the fetal heart is mentioned in Section 4.3. With experience, it may also be possible to identify Doppler signals from the placenta: they consist of a mixture due to movements at the fetal heart rate modulated by other movements at the maternal heart rate. During the last few weeks of pregnancy, an accuracy in placental localization of about 75 per cent was claimed in an early series [9.3]. More recently, one error in the estimation of the uterine segment containing the placenta was reported in a series [9.16] of 56 patients with definite confirmation of the placental site; and, in another series of 46 patients [9.4], an accuracy of 92 per cent was achieved. There is no doubt, however, that such excellent results cannot be expected without a great deal of experience in the method. It is particularly difficult to detect signals from a posterior placenta.

(ii) *Arterial flow*

The first application of the Doppler blood flow detector in the evaluation of arterial disease was simple in principle: the course of an artery was traced along the limb whilst the operator listened for sudden changes in the characteristics of the signal [9.29]. In the normal, the sound consists of two components superimposed on a continuous low-frequency signal. The first is high-pitched, and corresponds to systole, and the second is low-pitched, and occurs during diastole. Although the method offers a significant advantage in comparison with normal clinical methods in the diagnosis of thrombotic occlusions [9.27], non-occlusive clots, which are more likely to produce emboli, may be overlooked. When an artery is occluded, a collateral circulation develops. A crude test for the presence of a collateral circulation is the failure to detect a change in the distal flow signal when proximal compression is applied. Much more useful information may be obtained from measurements of the velocity-time waveforms recorded simultaneously at separate sites on the limb [9.40]. Usually the sites chosen are at the common femoral artery just below the inguinal ligament and the popliteal artery in the popliteal fossa, or the popliteal artery and the posterior tibial artery slightly above and behind the medial malleolus at the ankle. Three quantities can be determined. The first is the pulse *transit time* (T.T.) between the two measurement sites. The second is the *pulsatility index* (P.I.) at each site. This is defined as the sum of the maximum oscillatory energy of the Fourier harmonics of the Doppler frequency spectrum, divided by the mean energy over the cardiac cycle. The third is the *damping factor* (D.F.) between the two measurement sites, defined as the ratio of the P.I.s at the upstream and downstream sites.

An alternative and easier way of treating the data is to derive quantity P.I.', which closely approximates to the value of the pulsatility index. This is done by the use of a planimeter to obtain the integral (A) of the pulse waveform displayed on a sound spectrograph, corresponding to a complete pulse of duration T. Then:

$$P.I.' = |\hat{V}pk-pk|/\overline{V} \qquad (9.1)$$

where $\hat{V}pk-pk$ = peak forward velocity during the pulse, or difference between forward and peak reverse velocities if reverse flow occurs,

and $\overline{V}$ = $\int_0^T Vdt/T = A/T$

where V = velocity at time *t*.

In any individual patient, these indices can be used to grade arterial disease into one of four classes [9.10]. This is illustrated in Fig. 9.2.

The usual method of estimating blood pressure non-invasively depends on measuring the pressure required in a cuff to occlude arterial blood flow. There are various ways in which the arterial pulse distal to the cuff may be detected. The most common method is by a stethoscope placed over the artery. The Doppler motion detector is more sensitive, however, and is capable of sensing movements of the arterial wall which correspond to those heard on ausculation. Using ultrasound, it is possible to measure blood pressure in severely hypotensive patients, and in the newborn [9.18], where conventional methods may be difficult.

Blood pressure measurements made using the Doppler blood flow detector may also be of clinical relevance. The evaluation of *run-off* vessels in the arterial system in a limb may be made by measuring the cuff occlusion pressure at several segments along the limb, in the case of the arm with the ultrasonic probe either on the radial artery, or in the leg on the peroneal and tibeal arteries [9.1].

The continuous wave Doppler method provides a rapid and reliable indication of the patency of the vascular supply to a transplanted kidney [9.27, 9.32]. The ultrasonic probe is positioned on the abdominal wall, directly over the kidney. Diminishing flow velocity to an individual kidney warns that rejection is imminent.

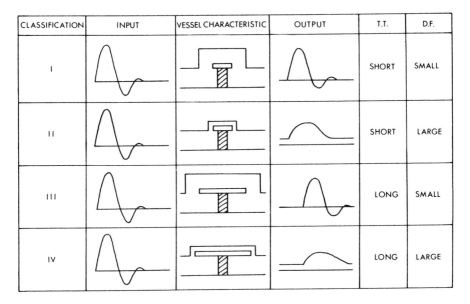

Fig. 9.2 Classification of arterial disease according to pulse transit time and damping factor. (The input and output waveforms show how the peak velocities measured from sound spectrograms change with time.) In physiological terms, these classifications correspond to (a) short, large diameter collateral; (b) short, small diameter collateral; (c) long, large diameter collateral; and (d), long, small diameter collateral.

Doppler signals arising primarily from blood moving in the thoracic aorta have been detected using a continuous wave 2 MHz Doppler system, the probe being placed in the suprasternal notch [9.24]. The orientation of the aortic arch is such that the ultrasonic beam intersects the direction of blood flow tangentially. Therefore, the highest Doppler shift at any instant corresponds to the highest velocity vector within the beam. The use of a real-time sound spectrograph to display directionally detected Doppler shift signals allows the operator to obtain optimal orientation, and to recognize flow signals from branch arteries which, since they serve the head and neck, are orientated so that the vector component of flow is in the opposite direction to that in the aortic arch. The spectral display allows turbulence to be identified, and can be interpreted even if the signal-to-noise ratio is poor.

The clinical usefulness of transcutaneous aortovelography is still being assessed [9.23, 9.25]. The part of the aorta in which the flow velocity is monitored is close to the heart, so that information on left heart action is obtained. In any particular individual, instantaneous cardiac output is likely to be proportional to the measured velocity, provided that the systolic cross-sectional area of the aorta, the velocity flow profile, and the fraction of flow in the branches of the aortic arch, all remain constant. Preliminary observations bear out the validity of these assumptions, and the method may be useful in critical care situations. The waveform of the envelope of the frequency spectrum also seems to reflect the cardiac performance in other respects, such as early systolic acceleration, peak velocity, and duration of acceleration and deceleration phases of the systolic period.

In blood flow studies, it is sometimes helpful to have a two-dimensional map showing the positions of blood vessels. In suitable anatomical sites—such as in the neck and the thigh—maps of this kind can be obtained by means of a two-dimensional scanner which plots the position of a Doppler probe. The Doppler probe is scanned over the patients's skin; where the ultrasonic beam intersects flowing blood, Doppler-shifted signals are detected which produce registrations on the storage display spatially related to the positions of the blood vessels. Venous and arterial signals can be distinguished by directional detection. Both continuous wave [9.35] and pulsed Dopplers [9.9, 9.31] have been used: the latter allow blood flows in the same directions, but spaced in range, to be separated, and can be used to plot cross-sectional images of the scanned vessels.

(iii)   *Venous flow*

Doppler signals from veins produce audible sounds which consist of a continuous rushing noise. Sudden compression of the extremity results in a distinct brief and high-pitched noise, called an 'augmented flow sound' [9.34]. Four such sounds may be elicited at any particular vein site. Two are normally heard, one associated with distal-compression, and the other, with proximal-pressure-release. Their absence indicates an occlusion. Sounds associated with distal-pressure-release and proximal-compression indicate incompetent deep venous valves.

A very simple technique may be useful in screening for deep vein thrombosis [9.7]. The Doppler probe is placed on the groin and the sounds from the femoral artery are detected. The probe is then moved 10–20 mm medially, until it lies over the femoral vein. Augmentation of the sound occurs when the calf (or the foot) is compressed if the circulation is patent. The method, for which a 2 MHz Doppler system is suitable, is superior to clinical assessment, and is most effective in detecting clots in the upper part of the limb. The radioactive fibrinogen test is complementary, being more effective in detecting thrombi in the calf.

Entire limbs can be explored to discover incompetent perforating veins, using a Doppler blood velocity detector [9.30]. The skin over the suspect area is marked with dots in a raster pattern, and the probe is placed normal to the skin over each dot in turn. At each position, the calf below the site, or the foot, is squeezed: if an incompetent perforator is present, the blood is heard to flow first in one direction, then in the other.

Right heart disease may result in specific changes in the jugular venous flow pattern as detected by a directionally-sensitive Doppler system [9.17]. In order to study this, the probe is placed behind the medial end of the right clavicle, with the patient lying on his back with his head slightly raised. Tricuspid regurgitation, and left-to-right atrial shunt, can be reliably detected in terms of venous return disturbances.

9.1.c. Detection of gas bubbles in blood

The occurrence of gas bubbles in blood (or tissue) is a well-recognized hazard in the decompression of divers and civil-engineering compressed air workers, in patients having extracorporeal blood circulation, and also in neurosurgical operations in which the patient is in the sitting position.

Three different methods have been used to detect such gas bubbles by ultrasound. Firstly, there is an increase in the attenuation of ultrasound caused by the presence of bubbles in tissue due to decompression, which may be observed with an A-scope, for example by the disappearance of the far-side echo with the probe placed on an ear-lobe [9.38]. Secondly, the increased attenuation due to gas bubbles in blood may be detected by a transmission method, for example with two transducers between which blood bypassed extra-corporeally is being circulated [9.26]. Thirdly, gas bubbles circulating *in vivo* give rise to characteristic changes in the output from a continuous-wave Doppler instrument (generally, 2 MHz systems have been used). Although this was first demonstrated with a probe implanted around the caudal vena cava in swine [9.11], in man it is customary to place the probe externally, usually on the chest wall over the heart [9.5, 9.6, 9.28, 9.29], or sometimes over the carotid artery [9.41]. The presence of gas bubbles in the blood is indicated by the occurrence, in addition to the usual Doppler signals, of a sound which resembles the high-pitched scratching of a gramophone needle sliding across a record [9.29]. These signals can easily be seen on an oscillograph display, and the method is extremely sensitive. Thus, it has been shown that the introduction of a little over 0·1 ml of air into the heart can be detected ultrasonically.

9.2. ENDOCRINOLOGY

9.2.a. Suprarenal glands

Suprarenal tumours may be difficult to detect by conventional diagnositc radiology. The normal suprarenal is seldom seen in two-dimensional ultrasonic scans in adults, but it can often be visualized in children, particularly on the left side [9.46]. Space-occupying suprarenal lesions in children can be quite reliably seen [9.42]. In adults, ultrasonic scanning is unlikely to demonstrate tumours of less than 30 mm diameter. The scan of a large tumour is shown in Fig. 9.3.

9.2.b. Thyroid gland

Examination of the thyroid gland by palpation and the use of radioisotopes is

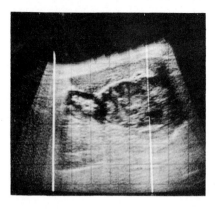
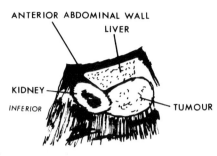

ANTERIOR ABDOMINAL WALL
LIVER
KIDNEY
INFERIOR
TUMOUR

Fig. 9.3 Suprarenal tumour. Longitudinal section, 60 mm right of midline.

generally satisfactory in the determination of the nature of thyroid lesions. Consequently, although the gland is readily accessible to ultrasonic investigation, it has not been the subject of extensive study by this method.

Preliminary results with a two-dimensional direct-contact B-scanner [9.43] have indicated that it may be possible to differentiate encapsulated and homogeneous adenomas from carcinomas. Rather encouraging results have been obtained with water-bath scanners producing both linear [9.44] and compounded [9.45] scans. Although the scan of the normal thyroid is relatively anechoic, its position may be localized by the relatively strong echoes from adjacent structures. Solid and cystic lesions can readily be distinguished [9.47], and proliferative lesions tend to give an increased echo density [9.44].

A water-bath scanner has been used to obtain two-dimensional B-scans from which the weight of the thyroid has been estimated [9.48]. This is complementary to scintigraphy, from which the functional volume may be found.

9.3   GASTROENTEROLOGY

Ultrasonic investigations of the liver, gall bladder, bile duct, and spleen, are discussed in Chapter 6. The present Section is concerned with the ultrasonic examinations of other structures in the gastrointestinal tract.

9.3.a.   Teeth and mouth

In the developed world, one of the main sources of exposure of the population to ionizing radiation is in the dental surgeries. Moreover, for the individual patient, the time required to process the films may involve delays and return visits. Therefore important advantages would be gained by the development of safe and rapid ultrasonic diagnostic techniques in dentistry, provided that the clinical results were as reliable as radiology and the apparatus was economical to purchase and to operate.

Both reflexion and transmission methods have been shown to be capable of detecting degenerative pulpitis [9.53]. Probes of 1 mm diameter were used, operating at 18 MHz. The transmission method depends upon the attenuation due to gas associated with pulpitis. It is more reliable than the reflexion method, because it is not affected by the inclination of the surfaces, but it does require access to both sides of the tooth.

The A-scope has been used [9.56] to study the positions of the dentinoenamel junction and the pulp chamber wall. A stand-off probe was used, with an aluminium rod (which has a similar characteristic impedance to that of dental enamel) positioned between the transducer and the tooth. The results of preliminary experiments showed that it may be possible to estimate the thickness of the water film between an amalgam filling and the dentine. It may also be possible to assess changes in the mineralization of the enamel [9.55].

A 15 MHz two-dimensional water-coupled B-scanner (of the type designed for examining the eye) has been used to visualize teeth [9.60]. Horizontal scans were made at 0·5 mm intervals. It was not possible to distinguish between fillings and caries.

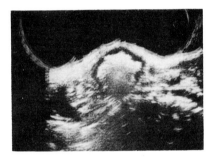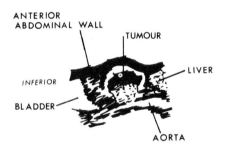

Fig. 9.4 Longitudinal midline section, showing carcinoma of the transverse colon. Note anechoic border region of the tumour, and dense echoes within.

It has been reported that it is possible to distinguish between solid and cystic lesions of the salivary glands by transcutaneous two-dimensional scanning through the upper neck [9.58].

9.3.b.   Stomach and intestine

Generally, ultrasonic scanning of some of the contents of the abdomen may be made difficult by the gas which tends to exist in the alimentary canal. At present, this often limits the clinically useful applications of the method in gastroenterology to the examination of the parenchymal organs of the upper abdomen, and the biliary system. There are a few exceptions. For example, it is possible to visualize omental cysts [9.59]. It has also been reported [9.5] that ultrasonic scanning can reveal bowel tumours as having almost non-reflecting outer layers with dense echoes from their centres. This is illustrated in Fig. 9.4.

9.3.c.   Pancreas

Investigation of the pancreas is a diagnostic challenge. A simple, safe and reliable method of examining the organ transcutaneously would be of great clinical value. At present, apart from ultrasound, there is no alternative to radiographic contrast study, x-ray tomography, or double-isotope scanning. Maybe computerized tomography will offer a solution, but its accuracy and cost remain to be determined.

The early attempts to examine the pancreas by ultrasound used the A-scope [9.62]; more recently, the two-dimensional B-scope, either direct contact or water coupled, has been used virtually exclusively. The frequencies have generally been in the range 2–3 MHz. The patient is examined in the supine position. Sometimes, better visualization of the pancreas can be achieved if the patient takes a mild laxative and fasts for 12 h before being scanned. Transverse scans are made close together to visualize the dorsal surface of the liver, the shadow of the stomach, and the anterior surfaces of the aorta and the vena cava. In the triangular space bounded by these three features, the portal vein is normally the only echo-free structure, and the head and body of the pancreas occupy most of the remaining volume; the tail lies behind the stomach and transverse colon. The full length of the pancreas can be seen in suitable individuals, displayed with the scan plane at an angle of about 20° to the transverse, caudally to the right. The mesenteric artery may be visualized just below this scan plane.

Instruments with bistable displays can be used reliably only to visualize the pancreas if it is enlarged by disease [9.49, 9.50, 9.52, 9.54]. The normal pancreas can often be visualized with gray-scale instruments, and the diagnosis of tumours, cysts and pseudocysts (see Fig. 9.5) can be quite reliable.

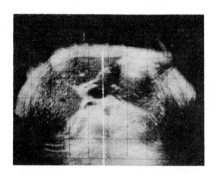 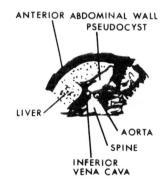

Fig. 9.5 Transverse section 40 mm below the xiphisternum, showing pancreatic pseudocyst.

When the nature of an enlarged pancreas is in doubt, ultrasonically guided fine needle biopsy may be helpful [9.51, 9.61]. Although the false negative rate is around 10–20 per cent, a positive biopsy confirming neoplasm may save the patient an unnecessary exploratory operation, since only 25 per cent of pancreatic cancers are resectable, and of these the 5-year survival rate is not better than 1 per cent.

9.4. ONCOLOGY

9.4.a. Ultrasonic scanning in radiotherapy and chemotherapy

Ultrasonic visualization of malignant lesions may be be of great clinical value in planning radiotherapy, and in assessing the effects of treatment, both by radiotherapy and by chemotherapy.

The high degree of accuracy which is potentially available with computerized planning in radiotherapy is not matched by the usual methods for obtaining data on patient contours and tumour location. Ultrasonic scanning has been used to provide images from which the radiotherapist, with the aid of a digitizing pen, can feed into a computer information including the surface geometry of the patient, and the locations of solid tumours and normal organs [9.64, 9.70, 9.75]. These data are stored in the computer, and may be displayed for subsequent amendment if necessary. Once the radiotherapist is satisfied that the information is accurate and complete, the computer is allowed to proceed with the preparation of the optimal treatment plan.

These methods have their most important applications in neoplasm of the retroperitoneal lymph nodes, the pancreas, the adrenals, the kidneys, the uterus, the ovaries, the bladder, and the prostate.

Direct observation by two-dimensional scanning of tumours treated by radiotherapy or chemotherapy is helpful in evaluating regression [9.63, 9.72, 9.73, 9.74]. If the regression rate is disappointing, the oncologist can cange the treatment schedule, or test the effect of different drugs.

Measurement of the thickness of the chest wall is helpful in planning electron beam radiotherapy (see Section 9.5.a).

9.4.b.   Investigations of the breast
Clinical examination of the breast is relatively easy; but doubt often arises about the nature of a breast lesion. This difficulty can generally be resolved by mammography. The major problem is to detect breast cancer at a very early stage, so that the possibility that earlier treatment may affect prognosis may be tested.

The breast is amongst the most accessible of structures to ultrasonic examination. Consequently, it was one of the first organs to be investigated ultrasonically, both by the A-scope at 15 MHz [9.78], and by 2 MHz [9.68] and 15 MHz [9.78] two-dimensional B-scopes. In retrospect, it is clear that the choice of such a high frequency as 15 MHz (with correspondingly rapid attenuation) seriously restricted the results, but it was demonstrated that malignant and non-malignant tissues could be differentiated ultrasonically. This distinction was made as the basis that the amplitude of echoes received from neoplastic tissue is statistically greater than that of those from the normal breast.

At frequencies of around 2 MHz, the diagnosis of cystic lesions is quite reliable [9.65, 9.66, 9.67, 9.77]. A typical scan is shown in Fig. 9.6. The appearances of solid lesions are less well delineated and defined than those of cysts. The identification of an abnormality is made easier if both breasts are shown on the same scan, so that any asymmetry is more obvious. It is apparent, from the literature [9.69, 9.71, 9.73], that non-compounded scans are often more easily interpreted than compound scans, even with gray scale. This is because some abnormalities can be recognized by the characteristics of the more distal echoes. Thus, lesions with relatively high attenuation are associated with lower amplitude distal echoes, and *vice versa*. The distal echoes in the former case are

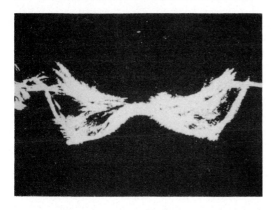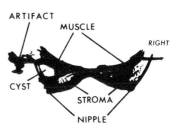

Fig. 9.6 Scan showing normal right breast, and cyst in left breast. Made using a water-immersion scanner operating at 2 MHz [9.77]. The artifacts which appear on both sides of the scan, but more markedly on the left, are due to reflexions at the water surface. (*Courtesy*: K.T. Evans.)

'shadows', and in the latter, 'anti-shadows'. Compound scanning masks this information by superimposing the shadows—or anti-shadows—over a wide arc of echoes from tissues surrounding the lesion.

One area in which ultrasound might have an impact on patient care, which does not seem yet to have been explored, is in the search for positive nodes in women known to have breast cancer. Almost 40 per cent may be missed by clinical examination. Their presence or absence is the most accurate indicator of the patient's prognosis: for example, when the nodes are negative, 80 per cent of patients survive at least 5 years. There is much controversy concerning the surgical approach, and whether or not a radical mastectomy is only necessary if the nodes are involved. Sooner or later this question will be resolved, and ultrasound may then have an important application in determining surgical strategy.

9.5. ORTHOPAEDICS AND RHEUMATOLOGY

9.5.a. Soft tissue thickness and oedema

The measurement of soft tissue thickness is chiefly important in two fields. Firstly, in anthropometry, ultrasound has been used to estimate fat thickness [9.80, 9.81, 9.90]. Secondly, ultrasonic measurements of soft tissue thickness have been used in the assessment of radiation effects on the lung [9.85, 9.88, 9.89]. Thus in electron beam radiotherapy, the treatment should be planned to avoid the hazard of radiation fibrosis in the lung. Similarly, the estimation by external detection of inhaled high-energy isotopes requires a knowledge of the soft tissue thickness of the chest wall.

Most investigators have used direct-contact probes, although some have used plastic rods [9.88] or water-filled balloons [9.89] to space the transducer from the skin to avoid the transmission pulse.

In the assessment of subcutaneous fat, the correlation between needle puncture and ultrasonic measurements in 100 individuals at a site 20 mm below and to the right of the umbilicus was 0·96 [9.81]. It is considered that the ultrasonic method is more accurate than Harpenden calipers [9.80].

The soft-tissue structures of the limbs, and particularly of the leg, may be demonstrated by ultrasonic two-dimensional scanning [9.82, 9.83, 9.84]. Generally, compound water-bath scanners operating at around 2 MHz have been used. The scans are capable of showing great detail, and are helpful in the assessment of oedema. Contact scanners may also be useful, and have been shown to be able to distinguish between Baker's cyst and thrombophlebitis [9.86], and to diagnose and assess popliteal cysts [9.87].

9.5.b. Assessment of fracture healing

The results have been reported of some preliminary experiments designed to test the possibility of assessing fracture healing in limbs in terms of the attenuation of shear waves transmitted across the fracture [9.83]. The rationale behind the method is that shear waves are rapidly attenuated in fluids so that the transmission of a shear wave across the region of a fracture is controlled largely by the extent of bone fusion, since liquid fills the space where fusion has not occurred. A somewhat similar technique has been proposed, based on changing transit time along the bone as the fracture unites [9.79]. Neither of these possibilities seems to have been given a clinical trial.

9.6. OTORHINOLARYNGOLOGY

9.6.a. Pharynx and vocal fold

Time-position recording has been used [9.94] to study the motion of the lateral pharyngeal wall during phonation. A 2·25 MHz ultrasonic probe is placed just below the angle of the mandible on the external neck wall. The technique may be useful in the evaluation of cleft palate patients prior to therapy, and in the rehabilitation of patients following laryngectomy.

A continuous-wave 6 MHz Doppler system has been used [9.95] to measure vocal fold motion during voice production. The probe is placed along the side of the neck immediately anterior to the oblique line of the thyroid cartilage at the level of the vocal cords. This non-invasive ultrasonic method gives results which are in good agreement with those obtained by high-speed ciné films.

9.6.b. Liquid collections

A 3 MHz A-scope has been used to detect the presence of liquid both in the maxillary sinus and in the middle ear [9.91]. In the first of these applications, a 10 mm diameter probe is held in contact with the skin on the face over the sinus. If the sinus contains liquid, an echo is received from its posterior wall; if it contains air, no such echo is received. Thus the ultrasonic technique should reduce the necessity to x-ray individuals, particularly children, suspected of having sinus problems. In the otological application, a smaller probe operating at a higher frequency is applied to the tympanic membrane.

9.6.c. Inner ear

The inner ear is normally inaccessible to ultrasonic examination, due to overlying bone and air. At the operation for the ultrasonic destruction of the labyrinth in Menière's disease and related disorders [9.92], however, a surgical approach is made towards the lateral semicircular canal. The surgeon aims to leave a bone thickness of about 0·5 mm over the canal, and it has been suggested that this could be measured by an ultrasonic pulse-echo technique. Preliminary experiments, using a 4 MHz probe, have given encouraging results [9.93].

9.7. RESPIRATORY DISEASE

9.7.a. Lung

In patients suspected of having pulmonary embolism, the diagnosis can usually be made clinically. It can generally be substantiated by scintigraphy. If this fails, pulmonary arteriography is only rarely thought to be advisable.

The interpretation of ultrasonic echoes obtained transcutaneously from lung is difficult because transmission is attenuated rapidly, whilst at the same time reverberation gives rise to artifacts. It has been reported that with a 2 MHz system, the length of the time-base on the A-scope occupied by echoes when the probe is in contact with the chest is much greater over areas of ischaemia than over normal lung [9.98]. This is probably due to decreased ventilation following interruption by pulmonary emboli in the perfusion of a lung segment [9.100]. A simple instrument has been developed with a 'yes-no' display and which generates an audible signal the pitch of which increases with increasing 'penetration' [9.96]. Using this device, it is apparently a simple matter to scan the lungs and thus to identify suspect areas.

9.7.b. Pleural effusion

The A-scope [9.99], the two-dimensional B-scope [9.101], and time-position recording [9.97], have all been used to demonstrate the value of ultrasound in the diagnosis of pleural effusion. The clinical problem is that the differential diagnosis of large opacities in a chest radiograph can be very difficult. In this situation, a liquid collection is anechoic and transonic, and ultrasound can delineate the anatomical structures, demonstrate the movement of the diaphragm, visualize liquid, and determine the best site for pleural tap. Thus the presence of a pleural effusion may be confirmed, and doubts about subphrenic collections and pleural thickening may be resolved.

REFERENCES

9.1. ANGIOLOGY

9.1. ALLEN, J.S. and TERRY, H.J. (1969). The evaluation of an ultrasonic flow detector for the assessment of peripheral vascular disease. *Cardiovasc. Res.,* **3**, 503–9.

9.2. BIRNHOLZ, J.C. (1973). Alternatives in the diagnosis of abdominal aortic aneurysm: combined use of isotope aortography and ultrasonography. *Am. J. Roentg.,* **118**, 809–13.

9.3. BISHOP, E.H. (1966). Obstetric uses of the ultrasonic motion sensor. *Am. J. Obstet. Gynec.,* **96**, 863–7.

9.4. COOPER, J.A., JOHN, A.H., ROSS, F.G.M. and DAVIES, E.R. (1969). Placental localization using an ultrasonic fetal pulse detector. *J. reprod. Med.,* **3**, 271–7.

9.5. EDMONDS-SEAL, J. and MAROON, J.C. (1969). Air embolism diagnosed with ultrasound. *Anaesthesia,* **24**, 438–40.

9.6. EVANS, A. and WALDER, D.N. (1970). Detection of circulating bubbles in the intact mammal. *Ultrasonics*, **8**, 216–7.

9.7. EVANS, D.S. and COCKETT, F.B. (1969). Diagnosis of deep-vein thrombosis with an ultrasonic Doppler technique. *Br. med. J.*, **2**, 802–4.

9.8. EVANS, G.C., LEHMAN, J.S., SEGAL, B.S., LIKOFF, W., ZISKIN, M. and KINGSLEY, B. (1967). Echoaortography. *Am. J. Cardiol.*, **19**, 91–6.

9.9. FISH, P. (1972). Visualising blood vessels by ultrasound. In *Blood Flow Measurement*, Ed. C. Roberts, pp. 29–32. London: Sector.

9.10. FITZGERALD, D.E., GOSLING, R.G. and WOODCOCK, J.P. (1971). Grading dynamic capability of arterial collateral circulation. *Lancet*, **1**, 66–7.

9.11. GILLIS, M.F., PETERSON, P.L. and KARAGIANES, M.T. (1968). *In-vivo* detection of circulating gas emboli associated with decompression sickness using the Doppler flowmeter. *Nature, Lond.*, **217**, 965–7.

9.12. GOLDBERG, B.B. (1971). Suprasternal ultrasonography. *J. Am. med. Ass.*, **215**, 245–50.

9.13. GOLDBERG, B.B., OSTRUM, B.J. and ISARD, H.J. (1966). Ultrasonic aortography. *J. Am. med. Ass.*, **198**, 353–8.

9.14. HOLM, H.H. (1971). Ultrasonic scanning in the diagnosis of space-occupying lesions of the upper abdomen. *Br. J. Radiol.*, **44**, 24–36.

9.15. HOLM, H.H., KRISTENSEN, J.K., MORTENSEN, T. and GAMMELGAARD, P.A. (1968). Ultrasonic diagnosis of arterial aneurysms. *Scand. J. thor. cardiovasc. Surg.*, **2**, 140–6.

9.16. HUNT, K.M. (1969). Placental localization using the Doptone fetal pulse detector. *J. Obstet. Gynaec. Br. Commonw.*, **76**, 144–7.

9.17. KALMANSON, D., VEYRAT, C., CHICHE, P. and WITCHITZ, S. (1974). Non-invasive diagnosis of right heart diseases and of left-to-right shunts using ultrasound. In *Cardiovascular Applications of Ultrasound*, ed. R. S. Reneman, pp. 361–70. Amsterdam: North-Holland.

9.18. KIRBY, R.R., KEMMERER, W.T. and MORGAN, J.L. (1969). Transcutaneous Doppler measurement of blood pressure. *Anesthesiology*, **31**, 86–9.

9.19. KRISTENSEN, J.K., HOLM, H.H. and RASMUSSEN, S.N. (1972). Ultrasonic diagnosis of aortic aneurysms. *J. cardiovasc. Surg.*, **13**, 168–74.

9.20. LAUSTELA, E. and TÄHTI, E. (1968). Echoaortography in abdominal aortic aneurysm. *Annls Chir. Gynaec. Fenn.*, **57**, 506–9.

9.21. LEOPOLD, G.R. (1970). Ultrasonic abdominal aortography. *Radiology*, **96**, 9–14.

9.22. LEOPOLD, G.R. (1975). Gray scale ultrasonic angiography of the upper abdomen. *J. clin. Ultrasound*, **3**, 665–71.

9.23. LIGHT, L.H. (1974). Initial evaluation of transcutaneous aortovelography—a new non-invasive technique for haemodynamic measurements in the major thoracic vessels. In *Cardiovascular Applications of Ultrasound*, Ed. R.S. Reneman, pp. 325–60. Amsterdam: North-Holland.

9.24. LIGHT, H. and CROSS, G. (1972). Cardiovascular data by transcutaneous aortovelography. In *Blood Flow Measurement*, Ed. C. Roberts, pp. 60–3. London: Sector.

9.25. LIGHT, L.H., CROSS, G. and HANSEN, G.L. (1974). Non-invasive measurement of blood velocity in the major thoracic vessels. *Proc. Roy. Soc. Med.*, **67**, 142–4.

9.26. MANLEY, D.M.J.P. (1969). Ultrasonic detection of gas bubbles in blood. *Ultrasonics*, **7**, 102–5.

9.27. MARCHIORO, T.L., STRANDNESS, D.E. and KRUGMIRE, R.J. (1969). The ultrasonic velocity detector for determining vascular patency in renal homografts. *Transplantation*, **8**, 296–8.

9.28. MAROON, J.C., EDMONDS-SEAL, J. and CAMPBELL, R.L. (1969). An ultrasonic method for detecting air bubbles. *J. Neurosurg.*, **31**, 196–201.

9.29. MAROON, J.C., GOODMAN, J.M., HORNER, T.G. and CAMPBELL, R.L. (1968). Detection of minute venous air emboli with ultrasound. *Surg. Gynec. Obstet.*, **127**, 1236–8.

9.30. MILLER, S.S. and FOOTE, A.V. (1974). The ultrasonic detection of incompetent perforating veins. *Br. J. Surg.*, **61**, 653–6.

9.31. MOZERSKY, D.J., HOKANSON, D.E., BAKER, D.W., SUMNER, D.S. and STRAND-NESS, D.E. (1971). Ultrasonic arteriography. *Arch. Surg.*, **103**, 663–7.

9.32. SAMPSON, D. (1969). Ultrasonic method for detecting rejection of human renal allotrans-plants. *Lancet*, **2**, 976–8.

9.33. SEGAL, B.L., LIKOFF, W., ASPERGER, F. and KINGSLEY B. (1966). Ultrasonic diagnosis of an abdominal aortic aneurysm. *Am. J. Cardiol.* **17**, 101–13.

9.34. SIGEL, B., POPKY, G.L., WAGNER, D.K., BOLAND, J.P., MAPP, E. McD. and FEIGL, P. (1968). Comparison of clinical and Doppler ultrasound evaluation of confirmed lower extremity venous disease. *Surgery, St. Louis*, **64**, 332–8.

9.35. SPENCER, M.P., REID, J.M., DAVIS, D.L. and PAULSON, P.S. (1974). Cervical carotid imaging with a continuous-wave Doppler flowmeter. *Stroke*, **5**, 145–54.
9.36. STRANDNESS, D.E., SCHULTZ, R.D., SUMNER, D.S. and RUSHMER, R.F. (1967). Ultrasonic flow detection. A useful technic in the evaluation of peripheral vascular disease. *Am. J. Surg.*, **113**, 311–20.
9.37. TAYLOR, K.J.W. (1975). Ultrasonic investigation of inferior vena-caval obstruction. *Br. J. Radiol.*, **48**, 1024–6.
9.38. WALDER, D.N., EVANS, A. and HEMPELMAN, H.V. (1968). Ultrasonic monitoring of decompression. *Lancet*, **1**, 897–8.
9.39. WINSBERG, F., COLE-BEUGLET, C. and MULDER, D.S. (1974). Continuous ultrasound 'B' scanning of abdominal aortic aneurysms. *Am. J. Roentg.*, **121**, 623–33.
9.40. WOODCOCK, J.P. (1970). The significance of changes in the velocity/time waveform in occlusive arterial disease of the leg. In *Ultrasonics in Biology and Medicine*, Ed. L. Filipczyński, pp. 243–50. Warsaw: Polish Scientific Publishers.
9.41. YAO, S.Y., NEEDHAM, T.N. and ASHTON, J.P. (1970). Transcutaneous measurement of blood flow by ultrasound. *Bio-med. Engng.*, **5**, 230–3.

9.2. ENDOCRINOLOGY
9.42. BEARMAN, S., SANDERS, R.C. and OH KOOK SANG (1973). B scan ultrasound in the evaluation of pediatric abdominal masses. *Radiology*, **108**, 111–7.
9.43. DAMASCELLI, B., CASCINELLI, N., LIVRAGHI, T. and VERONESI, U. (1968). Preoperative approach to thyroid tumours by two-dimensional pulsed echo technique. *Ultrasonics*, **6**, 242–3.
9.44. FUJIMOTO, Y., OKA, A., OMOTO, R. and HIROSE, M. (1967). Ultrasound scanning of the thyroid as a new diagnostic approach. *Ultrasonics*, **5**, 177–80.
9.45. JELLINS, J., KOSSOFF, G., WISEMAN, J., REEVE, T. and HALES, I. (1975). Ultrasonic grey scale visualization of the thyroid gland. *Ultrasound Med. Biol.*, **1**, 405–10.
9.46. LYONS, E.A., MURPHY, A.V. and ARNEIL, G.C. (1972). Sonar and its uses in kidney disease in children. *Arch. Dis. Child.*, **47**, 777–84.
9.47. RAMSAY, I. and MEIRE, H. (1975). Ultrasonics in the diagnosis of thyroid disease. *Clin. Radiol.*, **26**, 191–7.
9.48. TANAKA, K., WAGAI, T., KIKUCHI, Y., UCHIDA, R. and UEMATSU, S. (1966). Ultrasonic diagnosis in Japan. In *Diagnostic Ultrasound*, Ed. C.C. Grossman, J.H. Holmes, C. Joyner and E.W. Purnell, pp. 27–45. New York: Plenum Press.

9.3. GASTROENTEROLOGY
9.49. ENGELHART, G. and BLAUENSTEIN, U.W. (1970). Ultrasound in the diagnosis of malignant pancreatic tumours. *Gut*, **11**, 443–9.
9.50. FILLY, F.A. and FREIMANIS, A.K. (1970). Echographic diagnosis of pancreatic lesions. *Radiology*, **96**, 575–82.
9.51. HANCKE, S., HOLM, H.H. and KOCH, F. (1975). Ultrasonically guided percutaneous fine needle biopsy of the pancreas. *Surg. Gynec. Obstet.*, **140**, 361–4.
9.52. HOLM, H.H. (1971). Ultrasonic scanning in the diagnosis of space-occupying lesions of the upper abdomen. *Br. J. Radiol.*, **44**, 24–36.
9.53. KOSSOFF, G. and SHARPE, C.J. (1966). Examination of the contents of the pulp cavity in teeth. *Ultrasonics*, **4**, 77–83.
9.54. KRATOCHWIL, A., ROSENMAYR, F. and HOWANIETZ, L. (1973). Diagnosis of a traumatic pancreas cyst by means of ultrasound. *Ultrasound Med. Biol.*, **1**, 49–52.
9.55. LEES, S., GERHARD, F.B. and OPPENHEIM, F.G. (1973). Ultrasonic measurement of dental demineralization. *Ultrasonics*, **11**, 269–73.
9.56. LEES, S. and BARKER, F.E. (1971). Looking into the tooth and its surfaces with ultrasonics. *Ultrasonics* **9**, 95–100.
9.57. LUTZ, H. and RETTENMAIER, G. (1973). Sonographic pattern of tumors of the stomach and the intestine. *Excerpta Medica International Congress Series*, **277**, 31.
9.58. MACRIDIS, C.A., KOULOULAS, A., KOUTSIMBELAS, B. and YANNOULIS, G. (1975). Diagnosis of tumours of the salivary glands by ultrasonography. *Electromedica*, **43**, 130–4.
9.59. MITTELSTAEDT, C. (1975). Ultrasonic diagnosis of omental cysts. *J. clin. Ultrasound*, **3**, 673–6.
9.60. SMIRNOW, R. (1966). Diagnostic ultrasonics in dentistry. In *Diagnostic Ultrasound*, ed. C.C. Grossman, J.H. Holmes, C. Joyner and E.W. Purnell, pp. 300–5. New York: Plenum Press.
9.61. SMITH, E.H., BARTRUM, R.J., CHUNG, Y.C., D'ORSI, C.J., LOKICH, J., ABBRUZ-ZESE, A. and DONTANO, J. (1975). Percutaneous aspiration biopsy of the pancreas under ultrasonic guidance. *New Eng. J. Med.*, **292**, 825–8.

9.62. WAGAI, T., MIYAZAWA, R., ITO, K. and KIKUCHI, Y. (1965). Ultrasonic diagnosis of intracranial disease, breast tumors and abdominal diseases. In *Ultrasonic Energy*, Ed. E. Kelly, pp. 346–60. Urbana: University of Illinois Pres.

9.4. ONCOLOGY

9.63. BRASCHO, D.J. (1972). Clinical applications of diagnostic ultrasound in abdominal malignancy. *S. med. J.*, **65**, 1331–9.

9.64. BRASCHO, D.J. (1974). Computerized radiation treatment planning with ultrasound. *Am. J. Roentg.*, **120**, 213–23.

9.65. DAMASCELLI, B., MUSUMECI, R. and OREFICE, S. (1970). Sonar information about breast tumors. *Radiology.* **96**, 583–6.

9.66. DELAND, F.H. (1969). A modified technique of ultrasonography for the detection and differential diagnosis of breast lesions. *Am. J. Roentg.*, **105**, 446–52.

9.67. EVANS, G.C., LEHMAN, J.S., BRADY, L.W., SMYTH, M.G. and HART, D.J. (1966). Ultrasonic scanning of abdominal and pelvic organs using B-scan display. In *Diagnostic Ultrasound*, Ed. C.C. Grossman, J.H. Holmes, C. Joyner and E.W. Purnell, pp. 369–415. New York: Plenum Press.

9.68. HOWRY, D.H., STOTT, D.A. and BLISS, W.R. (1954). Ultrasonic visualization of carcinoma of the breast and other soft tissue structures. *Cancer, N.Y.*, **7**, 354–8.

9.69. JELLINS, J., KOSSOFF, G., REEVE, T.S. and BARRACLOUGH, B.H. (1975). Ultrasonic grey scale visualization of breast disease. *Ultrasound Med. Biol.*, **1**, 393–404.

9.70. JENTZSCH, K., KÄRCHER, K.H. and BÖHM, B. (1974). Ultraschall in der Strahlentherapie: bei der Bestrahlungsplanung und Überwachung des Therapiearfolges. *Ultrasound Med. Biol.*, **1**, 149–59.

9.71. KOBAYASHI, T. (1975). Ultrasonic diagnosis of breast cancer. *Ultrasound Med. Biol.*, **1**, 383–91.

9.72. KOBAYASHI, T., TAKATANI, O., HATTORI, N. and KIMURA, K. (1972). Clinical investigation of ultrasonographic patterns of malignant abdominal tumor in special reference to changes of its pattern after irradiation or chemotherapy (preliminary report). *Med. Ultrasonics*, **10**, 18–22.

9.73. KOBAYASHI, T., TAKATANI, O., HATTORI, N. and KIMURA, K. (1972). Clinical investigation of ultrasonotomographic patterns of malignant abdominal tumors in special reference to changes of its pattern after irradiation or chemotherapy. (II). *Med. Ultrasonics*, **10**, 132–5.

9.74. KOBAYASHI, T., TAKATANI, O., HATTORI, N. and KIMURA, K. (1974). Echographic evaluation of abdominal tumor regression during antineoplastic treatment. *J. clin. Ultrasound*, **2**, 131–41.

9.75. SLATER, J.M., NEILSEN, I.R., CHU, W.T., CARLSEN, E.N. and CHRISPENS, J.E. (1974). Radiotherapy treatment planning using ultrasound—sonic graph pen-computer system. *Cancer, N.Y.*, **34**, 96–9.

9.76. WAGAI, T., TAKAHASHI, S., OHASHI, H. and ICHINKAWA, H. (1967). A trial for quantitative diagnosis of breast tumor by ultrasonotomography. *Med. Ultrasonics*, **5**, 39–40.

9.77. WELLS, P.N.T. and EVANS, K.T. (1968). An immersion scanner for two-dimensional ultrasonic examination of the human breast. *Ultrasonics*, **6**, 220–8.

9.78. WILD, J.J. and REID, J.M. (1952). Further pilot echographic studies on the histologic structure of the living intact human breast. *Am. J. Path.*, **28**, 839–61.

9.5. ORTHOPAEDICS AND RHEUMATOLOGY

9.79. ABENDSCHEIN, W. and HYATT, G.W. (1972). Ultrasonics and the physical properties of healing bone. *J. Trauma*, **12**, 297–301.

9.80. BOOTH, R.A., GODDARD, B.A. and PATON, A. (1966). Measurement of fat thickness in man: a comparison of ultrasound, Harpenden calipers and electrical conductivity. *Br. J. Nutr.*, **20**, 719–25.

9.81. BULLEN B.A., QUAADE, F., OLESEN, E. and LUND, S.A. (1965). Ultrasonic reflection used for measuring subcutaneous fat in humans. *Hum. Biol.*, **37**, 375–84.

9.82. HOLMES, J.H. and HOWRY, D.H. (1958). Ultrasonic visualization of edema. *Trans. Am. clin. climat. Ass.*, **70**, 225–35.

9.83. HORN, C.A. and ROBINSON, D. (1965). Assessment of fracture healing by ultrasonics. *J. Coll. Radiol. Aust.*, **9**, 165–7.

9.84. HOWRY, D.H. (1965). A brief atlas of diagnostic ultrasonic radiologic results. *Radiol. Clin. N. Am.*, **3**, 433–52.

9.85. JACKSON, S.M., NAYLOR, G.P. AND KERBY, I.J. (1970). Ultrasonic measurement of postmastectomy chest wall thickness. *Br. J. Radiol.*, **43**, 458–61.

9.86. MCDONALD, D.G. and LEOPOLD, G.R. (1972). Ultrasound B-scanning in the differentiation of Baker's cyst and thrombophlebitis. *Br. J. Radiol.,* **45,** 729–32.

9.87. MEIRE, H.B., LINDSAY, D.J., SWINSON, D.R. and HAMILTON, E.B.D. (1974). Comparison of ultrasound and positive contrast arthrography in the diagnosis of popliteal and calf swellings. *Ann. rheum. Dis.,* **33,** 221–4.

9.88. RAMSDEN, D., PEABODY, C.O. and SPEIGHT, R.G. (1967). The use of ultrasonics to investigate soft tissue thickness on the human chest. *U.K.A.E.A. Reactor Group Report:* AEEW-R493. London: H.M.S.O.

9.89. ROSS, F.G.M. (1975). Ultrasound in diagnosis. In *Recent Advances in Radiology,* Ed. T. Lodge and R.E. Steiner, pp. 315–34. Edinburgh: Churchill Livingstone.

9.90. WHITTINGHAM, P.D.V.G. (1962). Measurement of tissue thickness by ultrasound. *Aerospace Med.,* **33,** 1121–8.

9.6. OTORHINOLARYNGOLOGY

9.91. BRZEZIŃSKA, H. (1972). Application of the ultrasonic echo method for laryngeal diagnostics in children. In *Ultrasonics in Biology and Medicine,* ed. L. Filipczyński, pp. 29–33. Warsaw: Polish Scientific Publishers.

9.92. JAMES, J.A. (1963). New developments in the ultrasonic therapy of Menière's disease. *Ann. Roy. Coll. Surg.,* **33,** 226–44.

9.93. JOHNSON, S., SJÖBERG, A. and STAHLE, J. (1966). Studies of the otic capsule. 1. Reduced dead time ultrasonic probe for the measurement of bone thickness. *Acta oto-lar.,* **62,** 532–44.

9.94. KELSEY, C.A., HIXON, T.J. and MINIFIE, F.D. (1968). Ultrasonic measurement of lateral pharyngeal wall displacement. *I.E.E.E. Trans. bio-med. Engng.,* **BME-16,** 143–7.

9.95 MINIFIE, F.D., KELSEY, C.A. and HIXON, T.J. (1968). Measurement of vocal fold motion using an ultrasonic Doppler velocity meter. *J. acoust. Soc. Am.,* **43,** 1165–9.

9.7. RESPIRATORY DISEASE

9.96. GORDON, D. (1974). A new ultrasonic technique for lung diagnosis. In *Ultrasonics in Medicine,* Ed M. de Vlieger, D.N. White and V.R. McCready, pp. 207–11. Excerpta Medica, Amsterdam.

9.97. JOYNER, C.R., HERMAN, R.J. and REID, J.M. (1967). Reflected ultrasound in the detection and localization of pleural effusion. *J. Am. med. Ass.,* **200,** 399–402.

9.98. MILLER, L.D., JOYNER, C.R., DUDRICK, S.J. and ESKIN, D.J. (1967). Clinical use of ultrasound in the early diagnosis of pulmonary embolism. *Ann. Surg.,* **166,** 381–92.

9.99. PELL, R.L. (1964). Ultrasound for routine clinical investigations. *Ultrasonics,* **2,** 87–9.

9.100.ROSS, A.M., GENTON, E. and HOLMES, J.H. (1968). Ultrasonic examination of the lung. *J. lab. clin. Med.,* **72,** 556–64.

9.101.TAYLOR, K.J.W. (1974). Use of ultrasound in opaque hemithorax. *Br. J. Radiol.,* **47,** 199–200.

PART III   BIOLOGICAL EFFECTS, INCLUDING
             THE POSSIBILITY OF
             HAZARD IN DIAGNOSTIC
             TECHNIQUES

10. Biological effects of ultrasound

C.R. HILL

10.1. INTRODUCTION

The generation of ultrasound in solids and liquids was first achieved in 1917 by the French physicist Langevin, who had the idea of using the piezoelectric effect to excite electrically a quartz crystal into mechanical oscillation at one of its resonant frequencies. The technique was rapidly developed in connexion with naval interest in echo-sounding and quite early in this work it was observed that small fish were being killed by the action of the sound beams. This observation was later confirmed by Wood and Loomis [10.44] in work carried out on fish, mice, unicellular organisms and blood, and subsequently by many other workers. It thus lead, in the 1930s, to a considerable interest in the possibilities for using ultrasound for tissue modification or destruction in a wide range of disorders, from cancer to *Violinspieler-Krampf* (Bergmann [10.1]). In retrospect, much of the work of this period may now appear naïve and partially to justify the subsequent reaction, that seems to have occurred in some quarters, against the use of ultrasound in medicine. From the comprehensive and critical survey of this period that is given by Bergmann [10.1], however, it is clear that the subject of ultrasound biology had already been shown to be of great interest although it undoubtedly suffered from the absence of a rigorous physical and quantitative approach.

A new phase in the medical and biological application of ultrasound commenced following the Second World War. On the one hand the military development of radar and sonar had provided the technology necessary for the introduction of pulse-echo techniques in diagnosis and, at the same time, the foundations were being laid for a quantitative, biophysical approach to the study of the biological effect of ultrasound. The latter owes much to the pioneering work at the University of Illinois by Fry and Dunn[10.14]. In spite of these developments, serious interest in the safety of medical ultrasonic procedures, and specific experimental investigation of the subject, date only from about 1964.

10.2. ULTRASOUND BIOPHYSICS

In order adequately to understand and interpret the large amount of experimental evidence now available relating to the 'biological effects of ultrasound', it is necessary to appreciate, at least in outline, the physical nature of the processes that occur when ultrasonic energy is absorbed by tissues and by experimental systems of interest to biologists. What follows is an attempt to summarize this subject, and necessarily omits much detail that can be found in the references. In this discussion it is implicit that the media of interest are liquids and soft tissues (which behave acoustically like liquids): in particular, except where specifically indicated, only longitudinal (*i.e.* compressional) wave motion is considered.

10.2.a.   Ultrasonic absorption

Attenuation of an ultrasonic beam by a medium occurs as a result of several processes which may be classified under the headings of true absorption, scattering and cavitation.

True absorption is a process that occurs at the level of inter- or intra-molecular organization and corresponds to the irreversible transfer of coherent mechanical energy to molecular or structural energy levels (see Section 1.1.f). Most, or all, of this energy ultimately appears as heat.

Ultrasonic absorption is a complex subject that is far from being fully understood even in simple media [10.2], and the further complexities that arise with biological media are very considerable [10.7, 10.41]. In a few very simple monatomic liquids absorption is due primarily to the viscous forces opposing mechanical movement of the medium but in molecular liquids, and particularly for large biological molecules, the predominant absorption mechanisms are related to inter- and intra-molecular structure. In living tissue it appears that absorption is due almost entirely to macro-molecules and a study on protein [10.25] has shown that a major part of the absorption is due to the rearrangement that occurs, under the action of oscillatory pressure, in the hydration shell surrounding the protein molecule. Since such rearrangement requires a finite time it tends to lag behind, and so to absorb energy from the pressure wave. It is not yet known whether so-called '*relaxation processes*' such as this can lead to any permanent modification of molecular structure other than that resulting from the thermal energy release to which they ultimately lead.

10.2.b.   Scattering

Ultrasonic scattering by tissues [10.20] is a subject that has been given very little attention hitherto, although evidence for its occurrence comes from observations of the return of diffuse echoes from macroscopically homogeneous tissue volumes in the process of ultrasonic pulse-echo diagnosis. Such scattering may arise from the existence in the medium of acoustic inhomogeneities (*e.g.*, density differences) and particularly those on a scale comparable with the ultrasonic wavelength (0.1—1 mm in tissue in the medical ultrasonic region). When an ultrasonic wave traverses such an inhomogeneous medium the different components vibrate with different amplitudes and thus move relatively to each other. It is this relative movement that is partly responsible for the scattering process, but it should be noted that not all the incident energy is reradiated: a significant fraction is absorbed by viscous forces.

Reliable information is not yet available as to the relative importance of this process of *inelastic scattering* as a contributor to overall attenuation but, for a number of soft tissues, it appears to be responsible for some 10 per cent of the total [10.20]. A further interesting aspect of this phenomenon is that relative oscillatory motion of tissue components can be expected, on theoretical grounds, to give rise to steady fluid streaming patterns within the tissue and, under certain experimental conditions, it has been shown that such streaming movement can lead to a variety of structural changes in cells and tissues [10.33].

10.2.c. Cavitation

The third attenuation process to be considered, *cavitation*, may be thought of as a form of scattering in which the scattering objects are themselves created by the action of the ultrasonic field. All normal liquids contain a considerable population of sub-microscopic gas bubbles and, under the action of mechanical vibration, these tend to grow by a process of *rectified diffusion* (net transfer of gas to the bubble from solution in the surrounding liquid). When such bubbles grow to a certain size in relation to the ultrasonic wavelength (about 6 μm diameter at 1 MHz) they behave as resonant cavities and their vibration amplitudes can become very large (several orders of magnitude greter than the vibration amplitude of the incident ultrasonic wave).

Such large amplitude vibration of bubbles within a liquid can lead, in two rather different ways, to modification of biological structures. In the first place, as in the case, noted above, of relative oscillatory motion occurring within tissue structures, the bubble vibration tends to set up a steady streaming pattern in the surrounding liquid, with consequent occurrence of localized high velocity gradients sufficient to shear cell membranes and large biological molecules [10.31]. In addition, however, as a result of the extremely rapid oscillatory compression of gas within the micro-bubbles, a phenomenon akin to ionization occurs in the gas volume and chemically highly reactive free radical species are produced and released into the surrounding liquid in high local concentrations. In this respect cavitation bears an interesting resemblance to ionizing radiation, and specifically to radiation of high linear energy transfer [10.40]. It has been shown that the rate of release of free radicals resulting from ultrasonic cavitation in water can be as high as that due to an absorbed dose rate of the order of 100 Gy min^{-1}.

The phenomena described above are sometimes referred to in the literature by the term *stable cavitation*, in distinction from *transient* or *collapse* cavitation, which is a phenomenon that generally only occurs at very high ultrasonic intensities and in which the liquid structure breaks down, giving rise to a cavity which collapses at the end of the negative half-cycle of the pressure wave [10.11]. In biology and medicine transient cavitation is only likely to be of significance under exceptional conditions of exposure but, as will be seen below, stable cavitation may play a major role at least in experimental studies involving liquid systems such as suspension cell culture. It should be emphasized that stable cavitation appears to be essentially a phenomenon of the liquid state and that there is no unequivocal evidence for its occurrence in organized mammalian tissues (although it has been observed in association with the small gas bubbles that are found in certain plant tissues). It is also relevant that the process of stimulation of stable cavitation, as described above, requires a finite period of time for its full attainment and thus, even in liquids, it does not occur in irradiations involving pulses of a few microseconds duration, relatively widely spaced, such as are used in pulse-echo diagnosis [10.19].

10.3. ULTRASOUND BIOLOGY

A very considerable volume of experimental work on the chemical and biological effects of ultrasound has been published in the past 45 years and it can, perhaps, best be classified in ascending order of complexity of the experimental system involved.

10.3.a. Chemical systems

The action of ultrasonically stimulated cavitation on simple chemical substances in aqueous solution has been studied by a number of authors and is reviewed elsewhere [10.10]. The effects here seem to be consistent with the action of the free radicals H and OH formed from water, but the precise nature of the reactions that occur is found to be dependent on the identity and concentration of gases dissolved in the water and thus capable of diffusing into the active cavities. A reaction that has been well studied, and is commonly used as an indicator of cavitation activity, is the release of free iodine from potassium iodide solution.

In addition to specific *sonochemical* action of this type, ultrasound is also capable of accelerating existing chemical reactions, such as the development of photographic emulsions [10.27], apparently as a result of the fluid stirring action that it induces.

10.3.b. Macro-molecules

Much attention has been given to the action of ultrasound on biological macro-molecules in aqueous solution and, in particular, to effects on DNA [10.32]. Here it is found that the primary effect is of a degradation process in which double strand breaks are induced and arise preferentially at the mid-point of the molecule, which suggests fluid shear as a causative mechanism. Although much of the work on this phenomenon has been done at low ultrasonic frequencies, in the region of 20 kHz, it has also been shown to be effective in the 0·25–4 MHz range at intensities of the order of 1 W cm^{-2} [10.10]. Evidence for free radical attack, based on observed changes in ultraviolet absorption and melting temperature in ultrasonically treated DNA solutions, has also been reported but this appears to be a relatively minor effect even in irradiations leading to very considerable degradation (*e.g.,* to a mean molecular weight of 0·25 million from an initial 10 million).

In general the mechanical and chemical effects are clearly attributable to cavitation, since they can be inhibited entirely by degassing the solution or by increasing the effective ambient pressure. It has been reported, however, that, at moderately high intensities (25 W cm^{-2} at 1 MHz), DNA can be degraded by a mechanism other than cavitation [10.16], although it has not been possible to detect degradation in proteins in the absence of cavitation [10.8].

10.3.c. Cells

Much of the early work on the biological effects of ultrasound was carried out on aqueous suspensions of micro-organisms or other single cells, and great interest in this type of system continues because of the compromise it appears to provide between biology and simplicity. The most commonly observed type of effect here is a catastrophic rupture of the cell membrane [10.22], and this in fact provides the basis for the action of the ultrasonic cell disintigrator [10.21]. The mechanism responsible for this effect is again cavitation and it has been shown that, although sonochemical action is normally present, its effects are likely to be buffered by the nutrient medium in which the cells are irradiated and it is thus, as with DNA degradation, the purely mechanical action of cavitation that is predominant [10.5]. Non-lethal damage to isolated cells, generally acting at the cell membrane, but possibly also at other sites, has also been demonstrated. Several experimenters, for example, have reported changes in the electrophoretic mobility of various mammalian cells apparently reflecting a reduction in the net surface electrical charge on the cell membrane, and this has been shown to be associated with the cavitational action of ultrasound, and also to be reversible [10.24]. A possibly related phenomenon is the observed increase in the permeability of certain cells to specific cytotoxic drugs, following ultrasonic irradiation of an *in vitro* suspension culture [10.26].

As noted above, cavitation is a phenomenon of the liquid state and it is doubtful whether it occurs in organized tissues. Thus, in attempting to understand the effects of ultrasound occurring at the cellular level in organized tissue, evidence from experiments on liquid suspensions of cells is of very limited value unless effective steps have been taken to inhibit cavitational action. Surprisingly little work has been attempted in this direction although it has been shown to be experimentally practicable, even for mammalian cells, for example by irradiating in gel suspension [10.6]. Another method of inhibiting cavitation is to use very short ultrasonic pulses and, by this means, it has been possible to study the response of the proliferation pattern of mammalian cells to ultrasonic irradiation and to show that no detectable change in this pattern is caused by irradiations for 5 h at a peak intensity of 15 W cm^{-2}, with pulses of 1 ms duration and duty factor 0·1 [10.4].

Microscopic observation of single cells undergoing ultrasonic irradiation has been carried out on large plant and marine egg cells, which are brought in close proximity to the tip of a needle vibrating at a frequency of about 20 kHz. Under these conditions, acoustic streaming of nucleoplasm and cytoplasm is seen to occur, with movement, deformation and eventual fragmentation of some intracellular bodies [10.42]. The irradiation fields employed in this work, however, differ from those typical of an ultrasonic beam in that they are very non-uniform, and it is uncertain to what extent similar effects may occur under uniform beam conditions, and at the considerably higher ultrasonic frequencies used in medical diagnostic applications.

It is of interest that changes in the visco-elastic properties of plant cell cytoplasm have been observed following beam irradiations at intensities less than 40 mW cm^{-2} at 1 MHz [10.23].

10.3.d.   Tissues

A central interest in ultrasound biology is the effects that take place in organized tissue, but it is just in this area that, up till now, interpretation of experimental data has been particularly difficult.

Two characteristics in which organized tissues differ appreciably from the simpler systems considered above are a relatively high ultrasonic absorption coefficient and relatively low thermal mobility (*i.e.*, low conductivity and zero convection). Thus temperature rise becomes an important consideration and, in practice, is a mode of action that can readily lead to modification or destruction of tissue function. It seems likely that this provides part of the basis for the therapeutic effectiveness that is claimed for ultrasound in physical medicine and it has been applied specifically in techniques, based on focused ultrasonic beams, for the destruction of small deep localized regions of tissue [10.13].

Another situation in which localized heating can become significant, and inadvertently so, occurs when an ultrasonic beam is incident on an interface between soft tissue and bone. In this case it is possible for an appreciable fraction of the beam energy to be radiated into soft tissue in the form of transverse vibrations, for which the absorption coefficient in soft tissue (and thus the local rate of heat deposition) may be several orders of magnitude greater than that applicable to the more common longitudinal vibrations.

Whilst such temperature effects can evidently be of great importance in some situations, a potentially much more interesting field of study has arisen from the demonstration that other, non-thermal and non-cavitational mechanisms of action of ultrasound can be effective in organized tissue. The first clear evidence for such a phenomenon was obtained in an experimental series of irradiations of mouse spinal cord, in which hind leg paralysis was used as an end-point [10.13]. It was shown that paralysis could be obtained in conditions where neither temperature rise nor cavitation were significant factors; and a potentiating effect was also demonstrated, in which paralysis followed from two exposures well separated in time, neither of which would be effective separately. Unfortunately, these early results were not thoroughly followed up at the time, but some more recent work [10.37] appears to confirm the general pattern of a threshold of accumulated exposure time, again with evidence against a thermal mechanism. Further support for this latter finding comes from a study on rat liver subjected to pulsed irradiation, in which marked qualitative differences in the lesions produced were found for different pulsing regimes but constant average exposure, and thus constant thermal effectiveness [10.36].

The effects contributing to the above observations all appear to be biologically destructive in their nature, and are thus in contrast with the demonstration of a significant increase in the rate of wound healing following low-intensity irradiation under conditions in which a thermal explanation can be discounted and cavitation is most improbable [10.9]. An enhanced rate of synthesis of DNA, and possibly also of protein, has been demonstrated in the regenerating tissues following treatment with ultrasound. It has been suggested that induced microstreaming movements in tissue fluid may be the physical mechanism responsible for these effects, but another interesting possibility is that they may result from the activity of enzymes released following ultrasonically induced rupture of lysosomal membranes [10.15].

Another reported finding, which the original author believed might also have a non-thermal basis, is that ultrasound, applied as an exposure that is in itself ineffective, is capable of enhancing by a factor of 1·7 the tumour-therapeutic effectiveness of a given dose of x-rays [10.43]. The possibility of a synergistic effect of this type is supported by some other reports, but in a recent attempt to repeat the original experiments, using both *in vivo* and *in vitro* techniques, it was not possible to demonstrate significant evidence for such synergism under conditions in which temperature was maintained constant [10.6].

10.4. INVESTIGATIONS OF HAZARD

It is possible to distinguish three rather different but complementary approaches to the elucidation of the hazards that might be involved in medical application of ultrasound [10.18]. The general study of the biology and biophysics of ultrasound, as described above, should eventually provide a fundamental understanding of all the processes that could lead to clinically harmful eff cts. This, however, is clearly a long term approach and it is necessary, in the s orter term, to carry out specific empirical investigations in which certain bir ogical endpoints, such as fetal abnormalities in rats or mice, are examined n relation to exposure parameters typical of particular medical applications. The third approach is that of epidemiology: this is the study of groups of individuals who have been exposed to ultrasound for medical or other reasons.

10.4.a. Experimental investigations

A practical difficulty enountered in planning specific experimental investigations of ultrasound hazard is that of knowing what effect to look for. Experience from the field of the hazards of ionizing radiation is not necessarily of direct relevance here, although it is indirectly of great value to the extent that it suggests useful criteria and high standards of judgment for such work. Viewed in this light the corresponding work on ultrasound appears to be at an early stage of development.

The first study directed specifically towards the problem of hazard of diagnostic ultrasound was designed to look for histological changes in animal brain tissue [10.12], but subsequent work has been concerned mainly with the possibility of genetic changes or somatic mutation. A considerable, and somewhat perplexing, body of work has been reported on this subject. A recent critical review has concluded that, with the possible exception of certain extreme exposure conditions where significant heat shock may be induced, present evidence does not point to a high risk of genetic effects from medical ultrasound, and that current diagnostic procedures in particular are very unlikely to result in a genetic hazard [10.38]. This conclusion is supported by the results of recent systematic searches for genetic changes in yeast systems [10.39] and in mice [10.28], following ultrasonic exposures greatly in excess of those in normal medical use.

Whilst a number of other simila studies have been equally reassuring [10.18], it is important to note that some isolated, apparently contradictory findings have been reported, particularly in relation to induction of cytogenetic [10.30] and teratogenic [10.34] changes. Although these reports were preliminary in nature, because of their potential significance they have both stimulated rather widespread series of follow-up studies, including subsequent investigations by one of the original authors [10.29.]. These have produced uniformly negative results for the mammalian cell systems that have been studied [10.3].

10.4.b. Epidemiology

As is again clear from experience in the related field of radiological safety, the epidemiological approach to hazard of ultrasound is likely to be difficult and beset with pitfalls. Only one serious study in this category has yet been reported [10.17]—on 1114 apparently normal pregnant women examined by ultrasound in three different centres and at various stages of pregnancy. A 2·7 per cent incidence of fetal abnormalities was found in the group, which compared with a figure of 4·8 per cent reported elsewhere in a separate and unmatched survey of women who had not had ultrasonic diagnosis. In the former study, neither the time in gestation at which the first examination was made, nor the number of examinations, seemed to increase the risk of fetal abnormality. Valuable as such a study is in the absence of better data, the quantitative significance of its findings must be somewhat open to question and, in the long term, it will be highly desirable to conduct more extensive and statistically controlled studies, preferably on a prospective rather than retrospective basis. Plans to carry out at least one major study of this kind are already well advanced.

10.5. CONCLUSION

The study of the biological effects of ultrasound is still, after 50 years, in a rather primitive state. Of the several distinct mechanisms of action that can be identified, the thermal effect is the simplest and best documented although the actual processes underlying ultrasonic absorption in mammalian tissues are poorly understood. Cavitation constitutes a very effective mechanism of action in liquid systems under the conditions in which much of the published experimental work on ultrasound biology has been carried out, but its occurrence under conditions experienced in *in vivo* medical applications is doubtful. Finally, evidence is accumulating for the existence of effects that are neither thermal or cavitational: their actual nature is unclear, and there are no substantial data to indicate that they could constitute a hazard in the medical use of ultrasound. This latter conclusion has been uniformly supported, whenever the work has been carried out under conditions that have been shown to be repeatable and quantitatively significant, by the evidence of toxicological studies on genetic and related phenomena.

REFERENCES

10.1. BERGMANN, L. (1954). *Der Ultraschall.* Stuttgart: Hirzel Verlag.

10.2. BHATIA, A.B. (1967). *Ultrasonic Absorption.* Oxford Clarendon Press.

10.3. *British Journal of Radiology* (1972). Five papers on possible induction of chromosome aberrations by ultrasound. *Br. J. Radiol.,* **45,** 320–42.

10.4. CLARKE, P.R. and HILL, C.R. (1969). Biological action of ultrasound in relation to the cell cycle. *Expl. Cell. Res.,* **58,** 443–4.

10.5. CLARKE, P.R. and HILL, C.R. (1970). Physical and chemical aspects of ultrasonic disruption of cells. *J. acoust. Soc. Am.,* **47,** 649–53.

10.6. CLARKE, P.R., HILL, C.R. and ADAMS, K. (1970). Synergism between ultrasound and x-rays in tumour therapy. *Br. J. Radiol.,* **43,** 97–9.

10.7. DUNN, F., EDMONDS, P.D. and FRY, W.J. (1969). Absorption and dispersion of ultrasound in biological media. In *Biological Engineering,* ed. H.P. Schwann, pp. 205–332. New York: McGraw-Hill.

10.8.   DUNN, F. and MACLEOD, R.M. (1968). Effects of intense noncavitating ultrasound on selected enzymes. *J. acoust. Soc. Am.*, **44**, 932–40.
10.9.   DYSON, M., POND, J.B., JOSEPH, J. and WARWICK, R. (1970). Stimulation of tissue regeneration by pulsed plane-wave ultrasound. *I.E.E.E. Trans. Sonics Ultrason.*, **SU-17**, 133–40.
10.10. El'piner, I.E. (1964). *Ultrasound: Physical, Chemical and Biological Effects*. New York: Consultants' Bureau.
10.11. FLYNN, H.G. (1964). Physics of acoustic cavitation in liquids. In *Physical Acoustics*, Ed. W.P. Mason, vol. IB, pp. 57–214. New York: Academic Press.
10.12. FRENCH, L.A., WILD, J.J. and NEAL, D. (1951). Attempts to determine harmful effects of pulsed ultrasound vibrations. *Cancer, N.Y.*, **4**, 342–4.
10.13. FRY, W.J. (1958). Intense ultrasound in investigations of the central nervous system. *Adv. biol. med. Phys.*, **6**, 281–348.
10.14. FRY, W.J. and DUNN, F. (1962). Ultrasound: analysis and experimental methods in biological research. In *Physical Techniques in Biological Research*, Ed. W.L. Nastuk, vol. IV, pp. 261–394. New York: Academic Press.
10.15. HARVEY, W., DYSON, M., POND, J.B. and GRAHAME, R. (1975). The 'in vitro' stimulation of protein synthesis in human fibroblasts by therapeutic levels of ultrasound. In *Ultrasonics in Medicine*, Ed. E. Kazner, M. de Vlieger, H.R. Müller and V.R. McCready, pp. 10–21. Amsterdam: Excerpta Medica.
10l.16. HAWLEY, S.A., MACLEOD, R.M. and DUNN, F. (1963). Degradation of DNA by intense, noncavitating ultrasound. *J. acoust. Soc. Am.*, **35**, 1285–7.
10.17. HELLMAN, L.M., DUFFUS, G.M., DONALD, I. and SUNDEN, B. (1970). Safety of diagnostic ultrasound in obstetrics. *Lancet*, **1**, 1133–5.
10.18. HILL, C.R. (1968). The possibility of hazard in medical and industrial applications of ultrasound. *Br. J. Radiol.*, **41**, 561–9.
10.19. HILL, C.R. (1972). Ultrasonic exposure thresholds for changes in cells and tissue. *J. acoust. Soc. Am.*, **52**, 667–72.
10.20. HILL, C.R., CHIVERS, R.C., HUGGINS, R.W. and NICHOLAS, D. (in press). Scattering of ultrasound by human tissues. In *Ultrasound: its Application in Medicine and Biology*, Ed. F.J. Fry. Amsterdam: Elsevier.
10.21. HUGHES, D.E. (1961). The disintegration of bacteria and other micro-organisms by the M.S.E.-Mullard ultrasonic disintegrator. *J. biochem. microbiol. Technol. Engng.*, **3**, 405–33.
10.22. HUGHES, D.E. and NYBORG, W.L. (1962). Cell disruption by ultrasound. *Science, N.Y.*, **138**, 108–14.
10.23. JOHNSSON, A. and LINDVALL, A. (1969). Effects of low-intensity ultrasound on viscous properties of *Helodea* cells. *Naturwissenschaften*, **56**, 40–1.
10.24. JOSHI, G.P., HILL, C.R. and FORRESTER, J.A. (1973). Mode of action of ultrasound on the surface charge of mammalian cells *in vitro*. *Ultrasound Med. Biol.*, **1**, 45–8.
10.25. KREMKAU, F.W., KAUFMANN, J.S., WALKER, M.M., BURCH, P.G. and SPURR, C.L. (1976). Ultrasonic enhancement of nitrogen mustard cytotoxicity in mouse leukaemia. *Cancer, N.Y.*, **37**, 1643–7.
10.26. KESSLER, L.W. and DUNN, F. (1969). Ultrasonic investigation of the conformal changes of bovine serum albumin in aqueous solution. *J. phys. Chem.*, **73**, 4256–63.
10.27. KOSSOFF, G. (1962). Calibration of ultrasonic therapeutic equipment. *Acustica*, **12**, 84–90.
10.28. LYON, M.F. and SIMPSON, G.M. (1974). An investigation into the possible genetic hazards of ultrasound. *Br. J. Radiol.*, **47**, 712–22.
10.29. MACINTOSH, I.J.C., BROWN, R.C. and COAKLEY, W.T. (1975). Ultrasound and 'in vitro' chromosome aberrations. *Br. J. Radiol.*, **48**, 230–2.
10.30. MACINTOSH, I.J.C. and DAVEY, D.A. (1972). Relationship between intensity of ultrasound and induction of chromosome aberrations. *Br. J. Radiol.*, **45**, 320–7.
10.31. NYBORG, W.L. (1965). Acoustic streaming. In *Physical Acoustics*, Ed. W.P. Mason, vol. IIB, pp. 265–331. New York: Academic Press.
10.32. PEACOCKE, A.R. and PRITCHARD, N.J. (1968). Some biophysical aspects of ultrasound. *Prog. biophys. Chem.*, **18**, 186–208.
10.33. RAVITZ, M.J. and SCHNITZLER, R.M. (1970). Morphological changes induced in the frog semitendinosus muscle fiber by localized ultrasound. *Expl. cell. Res.*, **60**, 78–85.
10.34. SHIMIZU, T. and SHOJI, R. (1973). An experimental safety study of mice exposed to low intensity ultrasound (abstract). *Excerpta Medica International Congress Series*, no. 277, p. 28.
10.35. TAYLOR, K.J.W. (1970). Ultrasonic damage to the spinal cord and the synergistic effect of hypoxia. *J. Path.*, **102**, 41–7.

10.36. TAYLOR, K.J.W. and CONNOLLY, C.C. (1969). Differing hepatic lesions caused by the same dose of ultrasound. *J. Path.*, **98**, 291–3.

10.37. TAYLOR, K.J.W. and POND, J.B. (1972). A study of the production of haemorrhagic injury and paraplegia in rat spinal cord by pulsed ultrasound of low megahertz frequencies in the context of the safety for clinical usage. *Br. J. Radiol.*, **45**, 343–53.

10.38. THACKER, J. (1973). The possibility of genetic hazard from ultrasonic radiation. *Current Topics in Radiation Research Quarterly*, **8**, 235–58.

10.39. THACKER, J. (1974). An assessment of ultrasonic radiation hazard using yeast genetic systems. *Br. J. Radiol.*, **47**, 130–8.

10.40. WEISSLER, A. (1959). Formation of hydrogen peroxide by ultrasonic waves. *J. Am. chem. Soc.*, **81**, 1077.

10.41. WELLS, P.N.T. (1975). Absorption and dispersion of ultrasound in biological tissue. *Ultrasound Med. Biol.*, **1**, 369–76.

10.42. WILSON, W.L., WIERCINSKI, F.J., NYBORG, W.L., SCHNITZLER, R.M. and SICHEL, F.J. (1966). Deformation and motion produced in isolated single cells by localized ultrasonic vibration. *J. acoust. Soc. Am.*, **40**, 1363–70.

10.43. WOEBER, K. (1965). The effect of ultrasound in the treatment of cancer. In *Ultrasonic Energy*, Ed. E. Kelly, pp. 137–49. Urbana: University of Illinois Press.

10.44. WOOD, R.W. and LOOMIS, A.L. (1927). The physical and biological effects of high-frequency sound waves of great intensity. *Phil. Mag.*, [7], **4**, 417–36.

APPENDIX

Equipment for ultrasonic diagnosis

A.1. SELECTION OF EQUIPMENT

Once the decision has been made to obtain equipment for ultrasonic diagnosis, it becomes necessary to choose from the bewilderingly wide range which is available. For a very few clinical applications, almost any equipment of the appropriate type is suitable; but, much more often, success depends upon the use of an instrument with an adequate performance. The novice finds the selection of equipment particularly difficult, although the correct decision at this stage may be crucial in subsequent clinical practice.

Because of the complexity of ultrasonic systems, it is not possible to give any general rules to guide the buyer. It may be helpful, however, to mention the features which should be considered when deciding whether a particular instrument is suitable for specific clinical application. In addition to assessing the specification of the equipment, it may also be wise to determine:

(*a*) How reliable is the equipment, and what servicing arrangements are available from the supplier?

(*b*) How many operators are required to use the equipment clinically?

(*c*) Is the performance of the equipment adequately stabilized against electronic drifts?

(*d*) Can the equipment be used by relatively untrained personnel?

(*e*) Is a special room required?

(*f*) Is the equipment easily portable?

(*g*) Does the price include import duty if liable?

A.1.a. Pulse-echo systems

(i) *General considerations*
The following considerations apply to the selection of A-scope, two-dimensional B-scope, and time-position recording systems.

Display. What size is the display? How bright is it? Is the spot size acceptably small? What facilities are there for photography? Can the display be viewed and photographed simultaneously? If there is an electronic storage facility, is it adequate (does the stored image degrade; how is it erased)? Is the gray-scale performance satisfactory? Are shift controls provided? Are there controls for focus and astigmatism? Is there a graticule?

Transmitter. Is the output variable (if so, is the output control calibrated)? Is the pulse length variable? What is the pulse repetition rate (and is it variable)? Is the maximum ultrasonic intensity as low as possible (to minimise the possibility of hazard)?

Probe. What size is the probe? At what frequency does it operate? What is the frequency response (is the pulse length short)? Is the ultrasonic beam focused? Are special probes available? Can the probe be sterilized? If the probe is an array, is it of a convenient construction?

Receiver. What frequency bands are available? Is the gain adequate? Is the gain control calibrated? Can swept gain be applied (if so, can the rate and the region of operation be adjusted by calibrated controls, and can this information be displayed simultaneously with an A-scan)? Can the undemodulated signal be displayed? Can suppression be applied? What are the characteristics of the video amplifier (*e.g.* linear or logarithmic, with or without differentiation)?

(ii) *A-scopes*
Is the time-base variable? Is it calibrated in terms of distance? Can distance-markers be displayed? Can the time-base be delayed relative to the transmission time (to examine in detail part of the time-base corresponding to a group of deep structures)? Can the trace be inverted; are there facilities for simultaneous display of data from two probes used in various modes (useful in neurological examinations)?

(iii) *Two-dimension B-scopes*
What coupling method is employed (direct contact or through a water bath)? What area can be scanned? How versatile is the scanning system (in order to scan in any plane, five degrees of freedom are required)? Is the mechanical engineering adequate? If it is a real-time system with a manual probe, is the probe freely maneouvreable? Is the registration accuracy adequate? Is the system suitable for special investigation (*e.g.* fetal cephalometry)? Particularly in the case of water-bath scanners, how quickly can a scan be made (*e.g.* is real-time visualization possible)?

(iv) *Time-position recording systems*
How is the recording made (by ultraviolet recorder, by still camera, on an electronic storage tube, or on a paper chart recorder by means of an analogue converter)? Can the recording be calibrated in terms of distance and time? Are there facilities for recording other physiological data (*e.g.* ECG and PCG)? In the case of analogue converter, can the position of the time-gate and the measured echo be identified on an A-scope?

A.1.b. Doppler systems

(i) *General considerations*
What is the size of the probe? What is the operating frequency? Is the ultrasonic field geometry appropriate to the clinical application? Is the ultrasonic intensity as low as possible (to minimize the possibility of hazard)? Are special probes available (*e.g.* for fetal monitoring, catheter-mounted, or for peri-arterial application)? Is the gain adequate? Does the instrument produce an acceptable sound (is it loud enough, is it harsh or noisy, are earphones available)? Is it operated by mains or battery power?

(ii) *More complex instruments*

Is the system range-gated? Has it a directionally-sensitive detector? If the output is by zero-crossing counter, is this adequate for the clinical application? Is there a frequency spectrum analyser (if so, how quickly is the analysis performed)?

A.2. AVAILABILITY OF EQUIPMENT

There is an increasing number of manufacturers of ultrasonic diagnostic instruments. Most of those believed presently to be offering equipment are listed here. The addresses of the headquarters of the manufacturers are given; most companies have subsidiaries or agents in other parts of the world. No responsibility can be accepted for errors and omissions.

The list is preceded by a table which gives the abbreviation used for the various systems, and also the approximate UK prices.

System	Abbreviation	Price, £ 000
A-scope	A	1–3+
Automatic echoencephalograph	AM	1–2+
Two-dimensional B-scope	TDS	6–30+
Real-time B-scope	RT	5–60+
Time-position recorder	TP	8–15+
Simple Doppler system	D	0·2–2+
Complex Doppler system	CD	0·5–10+

Manufacturer	System
Advanced Diagnostic Research Corporation 2202 South Priest Dirve Suite 102 Tempe, AR 85282 USA	RT
Aloka Co Ltd 6-22-1 Mure Mitaka-shi Tokyo 181 Japan	A TDS TP D
Alvar Electronic 6 Bis Rue du Progres 93107 Montreuil Paris France	TDS

Manufacturer	System
CGR 13 Square Max Hymans 75741 Paris France	TDS
Corometrics Medical Systems Inc Wallingford, CT 06492 USA	D
Delalande Electronique 30 rue Henri Regnault 92402 Courbevoie France	D CD
Diagnostic Electronics Corporation Box 580 Lexington, MA 02173 USA	AM RT
Diagnostic Sonar Ltd 35 Baron's Hill Avenue Linlithgow EH49 7JU UK	D
L'Electronique Appliquée 98 rue Maurice Arnoux 92120 Montrouge France	TP
Gruman Health Systems 400 Crossways Park Drive Woodbury, NY 11797 USA	RT
Hewlett Packard Inc 1501 Page Mill Road Palo Alto, CA 94304 USA	D
Hitachi Medical Coporation 1-1-14 Uchikanda Chiyoda-ku Tokyo Japan	D CD

Manufacturer	System
Kretztechnik GmbH	A
A-4871 Zipf	TDS
Austria	TP
	D
Litton Medical Systems	TDS
775 Nicholas Bvd	
Elk Grove Village, IL 60007, USA	
LKB Medical AB	A
Box 110	
161 11 Bromma, Sweden	
Mediscan Denmark	A
272 Kongevejen	TDS
2830 Virum	RT
Copenhagen	TP
Denmark	
Medishield Corporation Ltd	D
Hammersmith House	
London W6 9DX	
UK	
Metrix Inc	A
876 Ventura	TDS
Aurora, CO 80011	TP
USA	D
Nuclear Enterprises Ltd	A
Sighthill	TDS
Edinburgh EH11 4EY	TP
UK	
Nucleus Holdings (Pty) Ltd	TDS
5 Sirius Road	
Lane Cove	
New South Wales	
Australia	
Organon Technica BV	RT
Industielaan 84	
Oss	
Holland	

Manufacturer	System
Parks Electronics Laboratory 419 SW First Beavertron, OR 97005 USA.	D CD
Picker Corporation Medical Marketing Division 595 Miner Road Cleveland, OH 44143 USA	A TDS TP
Radionics Ltd 195 Graveline Street Montreal Quebec H4T 1R6 Canada	AM
Roche Bioelectronics Co Ltd 52 rue de Buzenval 92 St Cloud Paris France	RT CD
Rohé Scientific 2158 South Hathaway Street PO Box 10760 Santa Ana, CA 92711 USA	TDS
Searle Ultrasound 2270 Martin Avenue Santa Clara, CA 95050 USA	TDS
Siemens AG Medical Engineering Group Erlangen West Germany	RT
Smith Kline Instruments Inc 880 West Maude Avenue PO Box 1947 Sunnyvale, CA 94086 USA	A TDS RT TP D

Manufacturer	System
Sonicaid Ltd Hook Lane Nyetimber Bognor Regis, Sussex UK	D CD
Sonometrix Systems Inc 2067 Broadway New York, NY 10023 USA	TDS
Sophia 24 rue R. Valognes 78 Mantes-la-Ville France	CD
Techpan Swietokrzyska 21 Warsaw Poland	D CD
Toshiba 1–6 Uchisaiwaicho 1–chome Chiyoda-ku Tokyo 100 Japan	A TDS TP D
Unirad Corporation PO Box 39002 Denver, CO 80239 USA	A TDS TP
Varian Radiation Division 611 Hansen Way Palo Alto, CA 94303 USA	RT
Allen L. Wolff Co. 2485 Huntington Drive San Marino, CA 91108 USA	D CD

Index